Traditional British Recipes

© Copyright 2023. Laura Sommers.
All rights reserved.
No part of this book may be reproduced in any form or by any electronic or mechanical means without written permission of the author. All text, illustrations and design are the exclusive property of
Laura Sommers

- Introduction 1
- British Breakfast 2
  - Full English Breakfast 3
  - Porridge 4
  - Eggs Benedict 5
  - Kedgeree 7
- Main Courses 9
  - Roast Beef with Yorkshire Puddings 10
  - Fish and Chips 12
  - Cottage Pie 14
  - Bangers and Mash 16
  - Welsh Rarebit 18
  - Toad in the Hole 20
  - Shepherd's Pie 22
  - Steak and Kidney Pie 24
  - Lancashire Hotpot 26
- Desserts 28
  - Sticky Toffee Pudding 29
  - Eton Mess 31
  - Classic English Trifle 32
  - Chocolate Raspberry Trifle 33
  - Summer Berry Trifle 34
  - Apple Crumble 35
- English Afternoon Tea 36
  - English Black Tea 37
  - Cucumber and Cream Cheese Finger Sandwiches ... 38
  - Smoked Salmon and Cream Cheese Sandwiches 39
  - Smoked Salmon and Dill Finger Sandwiches 40

    Egg Salad Finger Sandwiches 41
    Roast Beef and Horseradish Finger Sandwiches 42
    Pesto and Tomato Finger Sandwiches 43
    Classic British Scones 44
    Fruit Scones 45
    Cheese Scones 47
Sweet Pastries and Cakes 48
    Mini Victoria Sponge Cakes 50
    Crumpets 51
British Snacks 53
    Homemade Crisps (Potato Chips) 54
    Digestive Biscuits 55
    Scotch Eggs 57
    Pork Pies 59
    Cornish Pasty 62
British Drinks 64
    British Earl Grey Tea 65
    Flat White Coffee 66
    Pimm's Cup 67
    Mulled Wine 68
About the Author 70
Other Books by Laura Sommers 71

Introduction

Welcome to a culinary journey that will take you through the rich and diverse flavors of British cuisine. This cookbook is a celebration of the time-honored traditions, the cherished regional specialties, and the cultural influences that have shaped the vibrant tapestry of British food.

Within these pages, you will discover an array of recipes that showcase the essence of traditional English cooking, from the comforting classics that have stood the test of time to the innovative creations that reflect the dynamic and evolving nature of the culinary landscape. From hearty breakfasts to elegant afternoon teas, from savory pies to delectable desserts, each recipe is a reflection of the culinary heritage and the warm hospitality that defines the British dining experience.

As you embark on this culinary adventure, you'll uncover the secrets behind iconic dishes like Fish and Chips, Yorkshire Puddings, and Shepherd's Pie. You'll be introduced to the art of brewing the perfect pot of British tea and savor the indulgence of traditional afternoon tea treats.

So, tie on your apron, gather your ingredients, and embark on a culinary adventure through the pages of this cookbook. Let the aromas, tastes, and textures of British cuisine fill your home, as you embrace the timeless traditions and embrace the vibrant spirit of British cooking. Let the journey begin!

British Breakfast

Breakfast in England is a cherished tradition, and the quintessential "Full English Breakfast" holds a special place in the hearts of locals and visitors alike. This hearty morning meal is known for its generous portions and diverse array of components. Typically featuring fried or poached eggs, bacon, sausages, grilled tomatoes, mushrooms, and black pudding, it provides a satisfying and filling start to the day. Baked beans in tomato sauce are another essential part of the breakfast, adding a touch of sweetness to the savory spread. Served alongside toast or fried bread, this classic breakfast is a celebration of comforting flavors and textures.

In addition to the iconic Full English Breakfast, England's breakfast culture extends to various regional specialties. For instance, in the coastal regions, you might find a "Seaside Breakfast" that includes locally caught fish such as kippers or smoked haddock. Meanwhile, further north in Scotland, you might encounter a "Scottish Breakfast," which features similar elements as the Full English but may include Scottish black pudding or haggis. In recent years, there has also been a rise in healthier breakfast options, with cafes and eateries offering avocado toast, porridge, and freshly squeezed juices to cater to more health-conscious diners.

Breakfast in England is not just about the food; it's also a social affair. Families and friends often gather around the table to enjoy a leisurely breakfast together, and many hotels and bed-and-breakfasts take pride in offering a traditional Full English Breakfast to their guests. Whether you opt for the indulgent classic or a lighter modern twist, breakfast in England is a delightful experience that sets the tone for a wonderful day ahead.

Full English Breakfast

A classic breakfast consisting of eggs, bacon, sausages, grilled tomatoes, mushrooms, black pudding, baked beans, and toast.

Ingredients:

Eggs (fried, poached, or scrambled)
Bacon (back bacon or streaky bacon)
Sausages (pork sausages or Cumberland sausages)
Black pudding (blood sausage)
Baked beans (in tomato sauce)
Grilled tomatoes
Grilled mushrooms
Toast or fried bread
Optional extras: hash browns, fried or grilled onions, fried tomatoes, bubble and squeak (fried leftover vegetables), and white or brown sauce

Directions:

1. Start by preparing the individual components of the Full English Breakfast.
2. Cook bacon in a frying pan or under the grill until crispy.
3. Cook the sausages in a separate pan until they are browned and cooked through.
4. In the same pan or a different one, cook the black pudding until heated through and crispy on the outside.
5. Heat the baked beans in a small saucepan over low heat.
6. Grill or pan-fry the tomatoes and mushrooms until they are cooked and slightly caramelized.
7. Prepare the eggs to your liking: fry them, poach them, or scramble them.
8. Optionally, you can also fry or grill some bread until crispy, or toast slices of bread.
9. Arrange all the cooked components on a large plate, and serve them together as a Full English Breakfast.

10. Serve with optional extras such as hash browns, fried or grilled onions, fried tomatoes, bubble and squeak, and condiments like ketchup or brown sauce.

Porridge

A warm, creamy dish made from oats, often served with milk and honey or sugar.

Ingredients:

1 cup rolled oats (old-fashioned oats)
2 cups water
1 cup milk (whole milk, almond milk, soy milk, or any milk of your choice)
Pinch of salt
Optional toppings: honey, maple syrup, brown sugar, fruits (e.g., sliced bananas, berries), nuts (e.g., almonds, walnuts), seeds (e.g., chia seeds, flaxseeds), and cinnamon or nutmeg

Directions:

1. In a medium-sized saucepan, bring the water and a pinch of salt to a boil over medium-high heat.
2. Once the water is boiling, add the rolled oats to the saucepan, stirring constantly.
3. Reduce the heat to medium-low and let the oats simmer in the water for about 5 minutes, stirring occasionally to prevent sticking.
4. After 5 minutes, add the milk to the saucepan, and continue to cook the oats for another 5 minutes or until the porridge reaches your desired consistency.
5. Stir occasionally to ensure even cooking.
6. For a thicker porridge, cook a bit longer.
7. For a creamier texture, you can add more milk or reduce the cooking time.
8. Once the porridge reaches your desired consistency, remove the saucepan from the heat.
9. Serve in bowls and add your favorite toppings such as honey, maple syrup, or brown sugar.
10. Add sliced fruits, nuts, seeds, and a sprinkle of cinnamon or nutmeg for added flavor and texture.

11. Stir the toppings into the porridge, and it's ready to enjoy!

Eggs Benedict

A luxurious breakfast consisting of poached eggs, Canadian bacon or ham, and hollandaise sauce served on toasted English muffins. It's a delightful and elegant way to start the day.

Ingredients:

4 large eggs
2 English muffins, split and toasted
8 slices Canadian bacon or ham
Fresh chives or parsley, chopped (for garnish)
For the Hollandaise Sauce:
3 large egg yolks
1 tbsp. lemon juice
1/2 cup unsalted butter, melted
1 pinch of cayenne pepper (optional)
Salt and freshly ground black pepper, to taste

Hollandaise Sauce Directions:

1. In a heatproof bowl, whisk together the egg yolks and lemon juice until well combined.
2. Place the bowl over a saucepan of simmering water (double boiler) and whisk continuously until the mixture thickens slightly.
3. Slowly drizzle in the melted butter while whisking constantly, until the sauce becomes smooth and thickened.
4. Be careful not to add the butter too quickly to avoid curdling.
5. Season the hollandaise sauce with a pinch of cayenne pepper (if using), salt, and freshly ground black pepper.
6. Keep the sauce warm by placing the bowl in a larger bowl of warm water.
7. Stir occasionally.

Poached Eggs Directions:

1. Fill a wide saucepan with about 2-3 inches of water and bring it to a gentle simmer over medium heat.
2. Add a splash of white vinegar to the water (this helps the eggs hold their shape).
3. Carefully crack each egg into a small bowl or ramekin.
4. Create a gentle whirlpool in the simmering water using a spoon. Gently slide one egg into the center of the whirlpool.
5. The swirling water will help the egg white wrap around the yolk.
6. Poach the egg for about 3-4 minutes for a soft and runny yolk or longer for a firmer yolk.
7. Use a slotted spoon to carefully remove the poached egg from the water and place it on a plate lined with paper towels.
8. Repeat the process with the remaining eggs.

Eggs Benedict Directions:

1. On each toasted English muffin half, place two slices of Canadian bacon or ham.
2. Carefully place a poached egg on top of the Canadian bacon or ham.
3. Spoon a generous amount of warm hollandaise sauce over each poached egg.
4. Garnish with chopped fresh chives or parsley for a pop of color and flavor.
5. Serve the Eggs Benedict immediately while still warm and the yolk is beautifully runny.
6. This delightful breakfast treat is perfect for a special occasion or a leisurely weekend morning, offering an indulgent and elegant way to start the day. Enjoy!

Kedgeree

A Delightful British Rice Dish. Kedgeree is a traditional British Rice dish with a fascinating history, originating from the colonial era when Indian spices were combined with British ingredients.

This flavorful and aromatic rice dish features smoked fish (often haddock), boiled eggs, and fragrant spices, creating a unique fusion of British and Indian flavors. Kedgeree is typically enjoyed as a hearty breakfast or brunch option but can also be served as a satisfying main course.

Ingredients:

1 cup long-grain white rice
2 cups water
1 lb.(450g) smoked haddock fillets (or any other smoked fish of your choice)
4 large eggs
1 large onion, finely chopped
2 tbsps. unsalted butter
1 tsp. curry powder (mild or hot, depending on preference)
1/2 tsp. ground turmeric
1/2 tsp. ground cumin
1/2 tsp. ground coriander
1/2 cup frozen peas
Salt and freshly ground black pepper, to taste
Fresh parsley or cilantro, chopped, for garnish
Lemon wedges, for serving

Directions:

1. In a saucepan, rinse the rice thoroughly under cold running water.
2. Add the rinsed rice and 2 cups of water to the saucepan.
3. Bring to a boil over medium heat, then reduce the heat to low, cover the saucepan, and let the rice simmer until cooked and the water is absorbed (about 15-18 minutes).

4. Once done, remove the saucepan from the heat and let the rice stand, covered, for an additional 5 minutes to steam.
5. While the rice is cooking, place the smoked haddock fillets in a separate pan and cover them with water.
6. Bring the water to a gentle simmer and poach the haddock for about 5-7 minutes until it is cooked through and flakes easily.
7. Once cooked, remove the haddock from the water, discard any skin and bones, and flake the fish into chunks.
8. In another saucepan, add the eggs and cover them with cold water.
9. Bring the water to a boil, then reduce the heat to a gentle simmer and cook the eggs for about 8-10 minutes until they are hard-boiled.
10. Once cooked, transfer the eggs to a bowl of cold water to cool. Peel and roughly chop the eggs.
11. In a large skillet or frying pan, melt the unsalted butter over medium heat.
12. Add the finely chopped onion and sauté until it becomes soft and translucent.
13. Stir in the curry powder, ground turmeric, ground cumin, and ground coriander, coating the onions with the aromatic spices.
14. Add the cooked rice, flaked smoked haddock, and frozen peas to the pan.
15. Gently fold the ingredients together until they are well combined and heated through.
16. Season the kedgeree with salt and freshly ground black pepper to taste.
17. Remove the kedgeree from the heat and garnish with chopped fresh parsley or cilantro.
18. Serve the kedgeree hot, with the chopped hard-boiled eggs on top and lemon wedges on the side for squeezing over the dish.

Main Courses

Main courses in England reflect a rich culinary heritage that combines traditional British dishes with influences from around the world. One of the most iconic main courses is the Sunday Roast, a beloved family meal typically served on Sundays. This classic dish features roasted meat, often beef, lamb, chicken, or pork, served with Yorkshire pudding, roasted potatoes, vegetables like carrots, peas, and broccoli, and lashings of rich gravy.

The Sunday Roast is a comforting and hearty meal that brings families together and is a staple in many British households.

Fish and Chips is another main course that holds a special place in English cuisine. This popular takeaway dish features battered and deep-fried white fish, such as cod or haddock, served with golden, crispy chips (French fries) and a side of mushy peas or tartar sauce. Fish and Chips have been a part of British food culture for centuries, with traditional "chippies" (fish and chip shops) found in every town and city across the country. It's a nostalgic and satisfying meal that is often enjoyed at the seaside or as a quick and tasty takeaway option.

In recent years, England has embraced global flavors, and its main courses have diversified to include a wide range of international dishes. Indian cuisine, in particular, has had a significant influence, with dishes like Chicken Tikka Masala, a spiced and creamy tomato-based curry, becoming a British favorite. Other popular international main courses include Italian pasta dishes like Spaghetti Bolognese and American-style BBQ ribs. This blending of cultures has enriched England's culinary landscape, offering a diverse array of main courses that cater to a wide range of tastes and preferences.

Roast Beef with Yorkshire Puddings

A Sunday roast featuring tender roast beef served with crispy Yorkshire puddings, roasted vegetables, and gravy.

Roast Beef Ingredients:

3 to 4 pounds (1.5 to 2 kg) beef roast (such as ribeye, sirloin, or top round)
2 tbsps. vegetable oil
Salt and freshly ground black pepper

Yorkshire Puddings Ingredients:

1 cup all-purpose flour
1 cup whole milk
2 large eggs
1/2 tsp. salt
1/4 cup beef drippings (reserved from the roast) or vegetable oil

Roast Beef Directions:

1. Preheat your oven to 425°F (220°C).
2. Pat the beef roast dry with paper towels. This helps to ensure a good sear on the meat.
3. Season the roast with salt and freshly ground black pepper on all sides.
4. In a roasting pan or a heavy oven-safe skillet, heat the vegetable oil over medium-high heat.
5. Sear the seasoned beef roast on all sides until it develops a nice brown crust.
6. Transfer the roasting pan or skillet to the preheated oven.
7. Roast the beef for about 20 to 25 minutes per pound (450g) for medium-rare or until the desired level of doneness is reached. Use a meat thermometer to check the internal temperature – it should read about 130°F (54°C) for medium-rare, 140°F (60°C) for medium, and 155°F (68°C) for medium-well.

8. Once the beef is done roasting, remove it from the oven and let it rest for about 15 minutes before slicing.

Yorkshire Puddings Directions:

1. While the beef is resting, make the Yorkshire pudding batter.
2. In a mixing bowl, whisk together the all-purpose flour, whole milk, eggs, and salt until you have a smooth batter.
3. Let the batter rest for about 30 minutes at room temperature.
4. Preheat your oven to 450°F (230°C).
5. In a muffin tin or individual Yorkshire pudding pans, add about a tsp. of beef drippings or vegetable oil to each cup.
6. Place the tin or pans in the preheated oven for about 5 minutes or until the fat is sizzling hot.
7. Carefully pour the Yorkshire pudding batter into the hot cups, filling them about two-thirds full.
8. Return the tin or pans to the oven and bake for approximately 20 to 25 minutes or until the puddings are puffed up and golden brown.
9. Remove the Yorkshire puddings from the oven and serve them immediately while they are still hot and fluffy.

Fish and Chips

Deep-fried battered fish (usually cod or haddock) served with chips (fries) and mushy peas.

Fish Ingredients:

4 white fish fillets (such as cod, haddock, or pollock) - about 6 oz. (170g) each
1 cup all-purpose flour
1 tsp. baking powder
1/2 tsp. salt
1 cup cold sparkling water or cold beer (sparkling water gives a lighter batter)
Vegetable oil, for frying

Chips Ingredients:

4 large potatoes, peeled and cut into thick strips (about the size of your index finger)
Vegetable oil, for frying
Salt, to taste

Chips Directions:

1. Rinse the potato strips under cold water to remove excess starch. Pat them dry with a clean kitchen towel or paper towels.
2. In a deep, heavy-bottomed pot or a deep fryer, heat vegetable oil to about 350°F (180°C).
3. Carefully add the potato strips to the hot oil in batches to avoid overcrowding. Fry them for about 5-7 minutes or until they are golden and crispy.
4. Remove the chips from the oil using a slotted spoon and transfer them to a plate lined with paper towels to drain any excess oil.
5. Sprinkle the hot chips with salt to taste.

Fish Directions:

1. In a mixing bowl, whisk together the flour, baking powder, and salt.
2. Slowly add the cold sparkling water or cold beer to the dry ingredients, whisking continuously until you have a smooth batter.
3. The batter should be thick enough to coat the back of a spoon but not overly dense.
4. Heat vegetable oil in a deep, heavy-bottomed pot or a deep fryer to about 350°F (180°C).
5. Dip each fish fillet into the batter, ensuring it is evenly coated.
6. Gently place the battered fish fillets into the hot oil and fry for about 5-7 minutes or until the batter is crispy and golden brown, and the fish is cooked through.
7. Remove the fish from the oil using a slotted spoon and place them on a plate lined with paper towels to drain any excess oil.

Serving Directions:

1. Serve the crispy Fish and Chips hot and immediately.
2. You can serve them with traditional accompaniments like malt vinegar, tartar sauce, or mushy peas.
3. Enjoy this classic British dish with a squeeze of lemon for a burst of citrusy flavor.

Cottage Pie

A savory pie made with minced meat (usually beef) topped with mashed potatoes and baked until golden.

Ingredients:

1 1/2 pounds (680g) ground beef (minced beef)
1 tbsp. vegetable oil
1 large onion, finely chopped
2 carrots, peeled and diced
2 cloves garlic, minced
2 tbsps. all-purpose flour
1 tbsp. tomato paste
1 cup beef broth
1/2 cup red wine (optional, can substitute with more beef broth)
1 tsp. Worcestershire sauce
1 tsp. dried thyme
Salt and pepper, to taste
For the mashed potatoes:
2 pounds (900g) russet potatoes, peeled and cut into chunks
1/4 cup unsalted butter
1/2 cup milk or heavy cream
Salt and pepper, to taste
1 cup shredded cheddar cheese (optional, for topping)

Directions:

1. Preheat your oven to 375°F (190°C).
2. In a large skillet or frying pan, heat the vegetable oil over medium heat.
3. Add the chopped onions and diced carrots and cook for about 5 minutes or until they soften.
4. Add the minced garlic and cook for an additional 1-2 minutes until fragrant.
5. Increase the heat to medium-high and add the ground beef to the pan.

6. Cook the beef, breaking it up with a spoon, until it's browned and cooked through.
7. Stir in the flour and tomato paste, coating the beef and vegetables evenly.
8. Pour in the beef broth and red wine (if using), stirring to combine.
9. Add Worcestershire sauce, dried thyme, salt, and pepper. Bring the mixture to a simmer and let it cook for a few minutes until the gravy thickens slightly.
10. Adjust the seasoning to taste.
11. While the beef mixture simmers, prepare the mashed potatoes. Place the peeled and cut potatoes in a large pot of salted water. Bring to a boil and cook until the potatoes are tender, about 15-20 minutes.
12. Drain the cooked potatoes and return them to the pot.
13. Add the butter and milk or heavy cream. Mash the potatoes until smooth and creamy. Season with salt and pepper to taste.
14. Transfer the beef mixture to a large oven-safe baking dish, spreading it evenly.
15. Spoon the mashed potatoes over the beef, covering it completely. Use a fork to create some texture on the surface of the mashed potatoes.
16. If desired, sprinkle shredded cheddar cheese on top of the mashed potatoes for an extra cheesy crust.
17. Place the Cottage Pie in the preheated oven and bake for 25-30 minutes or until the mashed potatoes are golden and the filling is bubbling.
18. Remove the Cottage Pie from the oven and let it cool slightly before serving.

Bangers and Mash

Sausages served with creamy mashed potatoes and onion gravy.

Ingredients:

8 pork sausages (traditionally Cumberland sausages)
2 pounds (900g) russet potatoes, peeled and cut into chunks
4 tbsps. unsalted butter
1/2 cup milk or heavy cream
Salt and pepper, to taste

Onion Gravy Ingredients:

2 large onions, thinly sliced
2 tbsps. unsalted butter
2 tbsps. all-purpose flour
1 1/2 cups beef or chicken broth
1 tbsp. Worcestershire sauce
Salt and pepper, to taste

Directions:

1. Start by preparing the mashed potatoes. Place the peeled and cut potatoes in a large pot of salted water. Bring to a boil and cook until the potatoes are tender, about 15-20 minutes.
2. While the potatoes cook, prepare the sausages. In a large skillet or frying pan, heat a little oil over medium heat.
3. Add the sausages and cook them until they are browned and cooked through, turning occasionally. This should take about 12-15 minutes.
4. Once the potatoes are tender, drain them and return them to the pot.
5. Add the butter and milk or heavy cream to the potatoes. Mash the potatoes until they are smooth and creamy. Season with salt and pepper to taste.

6. While the sausages and mashed potatoes are cooking, prepare the onion gravy. In a separate saucepan, melt the butter over medium heat.
7. Add the thinly sliced onions and cook them until they become soft and caramelized, about 10-15 minutes.
8. Sprinkle the flour over the onions and stir to coat them evenly.
9. Gradually pour in the beef or chicken broth, stirring constantly to avoid lumps.
10. Add the Worcestershire sauce, salt, and pepper. Bring the gravy to a simmer and cook for a few minutes until it thickens slightly.
11. Once the sausages, mashed potatoes, and onion gravy are ready, it's time to assemble the Bangers and Mash. Place a generous serving of mashed potatoes on each plate, top with sausages, and drizzle the onion gravy over the sausages.
12. Optionally, you can serve Bangers and Mash with a side of green peas or steamed vegetables for a complete and satisfying meal.

Welsh Rarebit

A savory dish made from a cheese sauce, usually served on toasted bread.

Ingredients:

2 tbsps. unsalted butter
2 tbsps. all-purpose flour
1 tsp. Dijon mustard
1 tsp. Worcestershire sauce
1/2 tsp. salt
1/2 tsp. black pepper
1/2 cup beer (such as ale or stout) or milk
2 1/2 cups grated sharp cheddar cheese
4-6 slices of bread (traditional choices include sourdough or a rustic white bread)

Directions:

1. In a saucepan over medium heat, melt the butter.
2. Stir in the flour and cook for about 1-2 minutes, stirring constantly, to form a roux.
3. Add the Dijon mustard, Worcestershire sauce, salt, and black pepper to the roux.
4. Mix well to combine.
5. Gradually pour in the beer (or milk), stirring constantly to prevent lumps from forming.
6. Continue stirring until the mixture thickens and becomes smooth.
7. Reduce the heat to low and add the grated cheddar cheese to the sauce.
8. Stir continuously until the cheese is completely melted and the sauce is smooth and creamy.
9. Be patient, as this may take a few minutes.
10. Once the cheese sauce is ready, remove the saucepan from the heat.
11. Toast the slices of bread until they are lightly golden and crispy. You can use a toaster or toast them under the broiler in your oven.

12. Pour the cheese sauce generously over the toasted bread slices.
13. Optionally, you can place the Welsh Rarebit under the broiler for a minute or two to give the top a golden and slightly bubbly finish.
14. Serve the Welsh Rarebit immediately while it's hot and bubbling.

Toad in the Hole

Sausages baked in a Yorkshire pudding batter until puffed and golden.

Ingredients:

8 pork sausages (traditionally Cumberland sausages or any other preferred sausage)
2 tbsps. vegetable oil
1 cup all-purpose flour
1/2 tsp. salt
3 large eggs
1 1/4 cups milk
1 tbsp. Dijon mustard (optional)
Freshly ground black pepper, to taste
2-3 sprigs of fresh thyme leaves (optional)

Directions:

1. Preheat your oven to 425°F (220°C).
2. In a large ovenproof baking dish, add the vegetable oil and place it in the preheated oven for about 5 minutes to get the oil hot.
3. While the oil is heating, prick the sausages with a fork in a few places. This will prevent them from bursting while baking.
4. Once the oil is hot, carefully remove the baking dish from the oven. Place the sausages in the hot oil, and return the dish to the oven.
5. Bake the sausages in the oven for about 10 minutes. This initial step helps to brown and partially cook the sausages before adding the batter.
6. While the sausages are baking, prepare the Yorkshire pudding batter. In a mixing bowl, combine the flour, salt, and black pepper.
7. In a separate bowl, whisk the eggs and milk together until well combined. You can also whisk in the Dijon mustard at this stage for extra flavor.

8. Gradually add the egg and milk mixture to the flour mixture, whisking continuously until you have a smooth batter.
9. You can add the thyme leaves to the batter at this point if using.
10. Remove the baking dish with the partially cooked sausages from the oven again.
11. Pour the Yorkshire pudding batter over the sausages, ensuring they are evenly covered.
12. Return the dish to the oven and bake for an additional 25-30 minutes or until the Yorkshire pudding is puffed up and golden brown.
13. Avoid opening the oven door during baking, as this can cause the Yorkshire pudding to deflate.
14. Once the Toad in the Hole is fully baked, remove it from the oven and let it cool slightly before serving.

Shepherd's Pie

Similar to Cottage Pie but made with minced lamb instead of beef.

Mashed Potatoes Ingredients:

2 pounds (900g) russet potatoes, peeled and cut into chunks
1/4 cup unsalted butter
1/2 cup milk or heavy cream
Salt and pepper, to taste
1 cup shredded cheddar cheese (optional, for topping)

Meat Filling Ingredients:

1 1/2 pounds (680g) ground lamb or beef
1 tbsp. vegetable oil
1 large onion, finely chopped
2 carrots, peeled and diced
1 cup frozen peas
2 cloves garlic, minced
2 tbsps. tomato paste
1 cup beef or chicken broth
1 tbsp. Worcestershire sauce
1 tsp. dried thyme
Salt and pepper, to taste

Mashed Potatoes Directions:

1. Place the peeled and cut potatoes in a large pot of salted water. Bring to a boil and cook until the potatoes are tender, about 15-20 minutes.
2. Drain the cooked potatoes and return them to the pot.
3. Add the butter and milk or heavy cream to the potatoes. Mash the potatoes until they are smooth and creamy. Season with salt and pepper to taste.
4. If desired, mix in shredded cheddar cheese for added richness and flavor.

Meat Filling Directions:

1. In a large skillet or frying pan, heat the vegetable oil over medium-high heat.
2. Add the chopped onions and diced carrots to the pan and cook for about 5 minutes or until they soften.
3. Add the minced garlic and cook for an additional 1-2 minutes until fragrant.
4. Push the vegetables to one side of the pan and add the ground lamb or beef to the other side.
5. Cook the meat until it's browned and cooked through, breaking it up with a spoon as it cooks.
6. Stir in the tomato paste, coating the meat and vegetables evenly.
7. Pour in the beef or chicken broth, Worcestershire sauce, dried thyme, salt, and pepper.
8. Mix well to combine all the ingredients.
9. Add the frozen peas to the meat mixture, stirring them in.
10. Let the meat filling simmer for a few minutes until the liquid thickens slightly.
11. Adjust the seasoning to taste.

Assembling and Baking Directions:

1. Preheat your oven to 375°F (190°C).
2. Grease a 9x13-inch baking dish or a similarly sized casserole dish.
3. Spread the cooked meat filling in an even layer at the bottom of the baking dish.
4. Spoon the mashed potatoes on top of the meat filling, spreading them to cover the filling completely.
5. Use a fork to create some texture on the surface of the mashed potatoes, which will help them brown nicely during baking.
6. Optionally, sprinkle some additional shredded cheddar cheese over the top of the mashed potatoes for an extra cheesy crust.
7. Place the Shepherd's Pie in the preheated oven and bake for about 25-30 minutes or until the mashed potatoes are golden and the filling is bubbling.

8. Remove the Shepherd's Pie from the oven and let it cool slightly before serving.
9. Chicken Tikka Masala: Although originally from India, this curry dish is widely enjoyed in the UK.

Steak and Kidney Pie

A hearty pie filled with tender steak and kidneys in a rich gravy.

Filling Ingredients:

1 lb (450g) beef steak, cut into bite-sized pieces
8 oz (225g) beef kidney, trimmed and cut into small pieces
1/4 cup all-purpose flour, for coating the meat
2 tbsps. vegetable oil or beef dripping
1 large onion, finely chopped
2 cloves garlic, minced
2 cups beef stock
1 tbsp. Worcestershire sauce
1 tbsp. tomato paste
1 tsp. dried thyme
Salt and freshly ground black pepper to taste

Pastry Ingredients:

2 1/2 cups all-purpose flour
1/2 tsp. salt
1 cup unsalted butter, cold and cubed
6-8 tbsps. ice-cold water

Filling Directions:

1. In a mixing bowl, toss the beef steak and kidney pieces with the all-purpose flour to coat them evenly.
2. In a large, heavy-bottomed pot or a Dutch oven, heat the vegetable oil or beef dripping over medium-high heat.
3. Add the coated beef and kidney pieces to the pot in batches, browning them on all sides. Remove each batch and set it aside.
4. In the same pot, add the chopped onion and minced garlic. Sauté them until softened and lightly browned.

5. Return the browned beef and kidney pieces to the pot, and stir in the beef stock, Worcestershire sauce, tomato paste, and dried thyme.
6. Season with salt and freshly ground black pepper to taste. Bring the mixture to a simmer.
7. Reduce the heat to low, cover the pot, and let the filling simmer gently for about 1 1/2 to 2 hours, or until the meat is tender and the flavors have melded together.
8. Stir occasionally.

Pastry Directions:

1. In a large mixing bowl, combine the all-purpose flour and salt.
2. Add the cold, cubed unsalted butter to the flour mixture.
3. Using your fingertips or a pastry cutter, rub the butter into the flour until the mixture resembles coarse breadcrumbs.
4. Gradually add ice-cold water, a tbsp. at a time, and mix the dough until it comes together.
5. Be careful not to overwork the dough.
6. Shape the dough into a ball, wrap it in plastic wrap, and refrigerate it for at least 30 minutes.
7. Assembly and Baking:
8. Preheat your oven to 375°F (190°C).
9. On a lightly floured surface, roll out two-thirds of the chilled pastry dough to fit the bottom and sides of a deep 9-inch (23cm) pie dish.
10. Fill the pie dish with the prepared steak and kidney filling.
11. Roll out the remaining pastry dough to create a lid for the pie.
12. Place the pastry lid on top of the filling and seal the edges by crimping them together.
13. Cut a small slit in the center of the pie to allow steam to escape during baking.
14. Brush the top of the pie with a beaten egg for a golden finish.

15. Bake the Steak and Kidney Pie in the preheated oven for about 30-35 minutes or until the pastry is beautifully golden and cooked through.
16. Remove the pie from the oven and let it cool slightly before serving.

Lancashire Hotpot

A one-pot dish with layers of meat (lamb or beef), onions, and potatoes, slow-cooked until tender.

Ingredients:

1 1/2 pounds (680g) boneless lamb shoulder or leg, trimmed and cut into chunks
2 tbsps. all-purpose flour
Salt and pepper, to taste
2 tbsps. vegetable oil
2 large onions, thinly sliced
2-3 large carrots, peeled and sliced
2-3 large potatoes, peeled and sliced
2 cups beef or lamb broth
2-3 sprigs of fresh thyme (or 1 tsp. dried thyme)
1 bay leaf
Butter, for greasing the baking dish

Directions:

1. Preheat your oven to 350°F (175°C).
2. In a large bowl, season the lamb chunks with salt and pepper. Sprinkle the flour over the lamb and toss to coat the meat evenly.
3. In a large, oven-safe casserole dish or Dutch oven, heat the vegetable oil over medium-high heat.
4. Add the floured lamb and sear it until browned on all sides. This will help to develop the flavors in the dish.
5. Remove the seared lamb from the casserole dish and set it aside.
6. In the same casserole dish, add a layer of sliced onions and carrots.
7. Place the seared lamb on top of the vegetables in an even layer.
8. Add another layer of sliced onions and carrots over the lamb.

9. Layer the sliced potatoes on top of the vegetables, arranging them in an overlapping pattern.
10. Season the layers with salt and pepper as you go.
11. Place the fresh thyme sprigs and the bay leaf on top of the final layer of potatoes.
12. Pour the beef or lamb broth over the ingredients in the casserole dish.
13. The liquid should come about two-thirds of the way up the dish; add more broth if needed.
14. Cover the casserole dish with a lid or aluminum foil.
15. Place the Lancashire Hotpot in the preheated oven and bake for approximately 2 to 2 1/2 hours, or until the lamb is tender and the potatoes are cooked through.
16. Remove the lid or foil during the last 30 minutes of baking to allow the top layer of potatoes to turn golden and crispy.
17. Once the Lancashire Hotpot is fully cooked, remove it from the oven and let it rest for a few minutes before serving.
18. Grease a plate or bowl with butter, then serve generous portions of the Lancashire Hotpot onto the plate.

Desserts

Desserts in England showcase a delightful array of sweet treats, from traditional classics to modern innovations. One of the most iconic and beloved British desserts is the Sticky Toffee Pudding. This moist and decadent sponge cake is made with dates and covered in a rich toffee sauce, often served warm with a scoop of vanilla ice cream or a dollop of custard. Sticky Toffee Pudding embodies the essence of comfort and indulgence and is a must-try for anyone exploring English desserts.

Another beloved dessert in England is the Eton Mess. This light and refreshing treat originated at Eton College and typically consists of layers of crushed meringue, whipped cream, and fresh berries, such as strawberries or raspberries. The combination of crunchy meringue, airy cream, and juicy fruit creates a harmonious medley of textures and flavors, making Eton Mess a popular choice during the summer months.

English trifle is a classic dessert that graces many tables during holidays and special occasions. This layered dessert features sponge cake soaked in sherry or fruit juice, custard, jelly (Jell-O), and fresh fruit, all topped with a generous layer of whipped cream. Trifle recipes can vary, and families often have their own cherished versions passed down through generations. With its vibrant colors and luscious layers, trifle is a show-stopping centerpiece that brings joy to dessert enthusiasts of all ages.

While traditional British desserts hold a special place in the hearts of many, England's dessert scene has also embraced contemporary influences. Dessert shops and patisseries offer a wide variety of modern treats, from artisanal cupcakes and macarons to innovative flavor combinations in ice creams and gelatos. Whether you prefer the nostalgia of a time-honored classic or the excitement of a cutting-edge creation, England's desserts promise to satisfy any sweet tooth.

Sticky Toffee Pudding

A moist sponge cake made with dates, covered in toffee sauce, and served with custard or ice cream.

Pudding Ingredients:

1 cup (200g) pitted dates, chopped
1 cup (240ml) boiling water
1 tsp. baking soda
1 1/2 cups (190g) all-purpose flour
1 tsp. baking powder
1/4 tsp. salt
1/2 cup (115g) unsalted butter, softened
3/4 cup (150g) granulated sugar
2 large eggs, at room temperature
1 tsp. vanilla extract

Toffee Sauce Ingredients:

1 cup (240ml) heavy cream (whipping cream)
1/2 cup (115g) unsalted butter
1 cup (200g) packed light brown sugar
1 tsp. vanilla extract

Directions:

1. Preheat your oven to 350°F (175°C). Grease an 8x8-inch (20x20cm) square or 9-inch (23cm) round baking pan.
2. In a bowl, combine the chopped dates and boiling water.
3. Stir in the baking soda and let it sit for about 10 minutes to soften the dates.
4. In a separate bowl, whisk together the all-purpose flour, baking powder, and salt.
5. Using an electric mixer, cream the softened butter and granulated sugar until light and fluffy.
6. Beat in the eggs, one at a time, followed by the vanilla extract.
7. Gradually add the dry flour mixture to the wet ingredients, mixing until just combined.

8. Fold in the softened dates along with any remaining liquid.
9. Pour the batter into the prepared baking pan and spread it evenly.
10. Bake in the preheated oven for 30-35 minutes or until a toothpick inserted into the center comes out clean.
11. While the pudding is baking, prepare the toffee sauce. In a saucepan, combine the heavy cream, unsalted butter, and light brown sugar.
12. Cook over medium heat, stirring constantly, until the mixture comes to a boil.
13. Reduce the heat and let the sauce simmer for about 5 minutes, stirring occasionally, until it thickens slightly.
14. Remove the saucepan from the heat and stir in the vanilla extract.
15. Once the pudding is done baking, poke several holes all over the top using a skewer or fork.
16. Pour about half of the warm toffee sauce over the hot pudding, allowing it to soak into the holes.
17. Let the pudding rest for a few minutes to absorb the toffee sauce.
18. Serve warm, drizzled with additional toffee sauce, and optionally, with a scoop of vanilla ice cream or a dollop of whipped cream.

Eton Mess

A delightful dessert made with crushed meringue, whipped cream, and fresh strawberries.

Ingredients:

4 large meringue nests, broken into small pieces
2 cups heavy cream (whipping cream)
2 tbsps. powdered sugar (icing sugar)
1 tsp. vanilla extract
2 cups mixed fresh berries (strawberries, raspberries, blueberries, or any berries of your choice)

Optional Ingredients:

Sprigs of fresh mint for garnish

Directions:

1. In a large mixing bowl, whip the heavy cream with an electric mixer until it forms soft peaks.
2. Add the powdered sugar and vanilla extract to the whipped cream and continue to whip until it forms stiff peaks.
3. Be careful not to over-whip the cream.
4. Gently fold the broken meringue pieces into the whipped cream until well combined.
5. The meringue should be partially crushed, creating a mixture of different textures.
6. Add about half of the fresh berries to the cream and meringue mixture.
7. Gently fold them in, allowing the berries to slightly crush and release their juices, creating streaks of color throughout the dessert.
8. Reserve some whole berries for garnishing.
9. Spoon the Eton Mess mixture into serving glasses or a large serving bowl.
10. Top the dessert with the remaining fresh berries and garnish with a few sprigs of fresh mint if desired.

11. Serve immediately, as the meringue will soften over time due to the moisture from the berries and cream.

Classic English Trifle

Layers of sponge cake, fruit, jelly, custard, and whipped cream, chilled to perfection.

Ingredients:

1 store-bought or homemade sponge cake or pound cake, cut into cubes
1/4 cup sherry or fruit juice (such as orange juice)
1 cup fresh mixed berries (strawberries, blueberries, raspberries)
1 cup vanilla custard (store-bought or homemade)
1 cup whipped cream
Slivered almonds or grated chocolate for garnish

Directions:

1. In a trifle dish or a large glass bowl, arrange a layer of sponge cake cubes at the bottom.
2. Drizzle the sherry or fruit juice over the cake cubes, allowing it to soak in.
3. Add a layer of mixed berries over the cake.
4. Spoon a layer of vanilla custard on top of the berries.
5. Repeat the layers until you have used up all the ingredients, ending with a layer of whipped cream.
6. Garnish the trifle with slivered almonds or grated chocolate.
7. Refrigerate the trifle for at least 2 hours or overnight before serving, allowing the flavors to meld together.

Chocolate Raspberry Trifle

Ingredients:

1 chocolate cake, baked and cooled, cut into cubes
1 cup raspberry jam
1 cup fresh raspberries
1 cup chocolate pudding (store-bought or homemade)
1 cup whipped cream
Chocolate shavings or cocoa powder for garnish

Directions:

1. In a trifle dish or a large glass bowl, layer half of the chocolate cake cubes at the bottom.
2. Spread a layer of raspberry jam over the cake cubes.
3. Add a layer of fresh raspberries on top of the jam.
4. Spoon a layer of chocolate pudding over the raspberries.
5. Repeat the layers with the remaining cake, jam, raspberries, and chocolate pudding.
6. Top the trifle with whipped cream and garnish with chocolate shavings or a dusting of cocoa powder.
7. Refrigerate the trifle for at least 2 hours before serving to allow the flavors to meld together.

Summer Berry Trifle

Ingredients:

1 store-bought or homemade angel food cake, cut into cubes
1/2 cup orange juice or berry-flavored liqueur (optional)
2 cups mixed fresh berries (strawberries, blueberries, blackberries, raspberries)
1 cup lemon curd (store-bought or homemade)
1 cup whipped cream
Fresh mint leaves for garnish

Directions:

1. In a trifle dish or a large glass bowl, arrange a layer of angel food cake cubes at the bottom.
2. Drizzle the orange juice or berry-flavored liqueur (if using) over the cake cubes.
3. Add a layer of mixed fresh berries over the cake.
4. Spoon a layer of lemon curd on top of the berries.
5. Repeat the layers until you have used up all the ingredients, ending with a layer of whipped cream.
6. Garnish the trifle with fresh mint leaves.
7. Refrigerate the trifle for at least 2 hours or overnight before serving to allow the flavors to meld together.

Apple Crumble

Baked apples with a crumbly topping of flour, sugar, and butter, served with custard or ice cream.

Apple Filling Ingredients:

4 large apples (such as Granny Smith or Bramley), peeled, cored, and sliced
1/4 cup granulated sugar
1 tbsp. lemon juice
1 tsp. ground cinnamon
1/4 tsp. ground nutmeg

Crumble Topping Ingredients:

1 cup all-purpose flour
1/2 cup rolled oats
1/2 cup packed light brown sugar
1/2 cup unsalted butter, cold and cubed

Directions:

1. Preheat your oven to 375°F (190°C). Grease a 9-inch (23cm) baking dish or pie dish.
2. In a bowl, toss the sliced apples with the granulated sugar, lemon juice, ground cinnamon, and ground nutmeg until well coated.
3. Spread the apple mixture evenly in the greased baking dish.
4. In a separate bowl, combine the all-purpose flour, rolled oats, and packed light brown sugar for the crumble topping.
5. Add the cold, cubed unsalted butter to the dry ingredients and use your fingers or a pastry cutter to rub the butter into the flour mixture until it resembles coarse crumbs.
6. Sprinkle the crumble topping evenly over the apple filling in the baking dish.
7. Bake for about 35-40 minutes or until the topping is golden brown, and the apple filling is bubbly and tender.
8. Remove from oven and let cool slightly before serving.

English Afternoon Tea

The quintessential British tradition involves tea served with finger sandwiches, scones, and pastries.

Afternoon tea is an enduring and cherished tradition in England, steeped in elegance and culinary delights. Dating back to the early 19th century, this quintessential British ritual is an invitation to pause, connect, and savor a moment of refined indulgence. Set in ornate tearooms, historic hotels, or even the comfort of one's home, afternoon tea offers a delightful spread of finger sandwiches, freshly baked scones with clotted cream and jam, and an array of dainty pastries and cakes.

Beyond its delectable treats, afternoon tea embodies the essence of British hospitality and camaraderie. It provides an opportunity for friends and family to gather, converse, and create cherished memories over a pot of perfectly brewed tea.
The act of pouring tea from elegant china teapots and using delicate teacups adds a touch of sophistication to the experience.

Through the generations, afternoon tea has retained its allure, evolving to incorporate modern twists and creative variations while remaining true to its roots. Today, it continues to be a celebrated tradition, offering a respite from the hustle and bustle of everyday life and inviting all to partake in a timeless ritual of charm, sophistication, and, of course, scrumptious treats.

English Black Tea

English Tea, often simply referred to as "a cuppa," is a beloved British beverage that is both comforting and refreshing. This classic black tea is typically served with a splash of milk, but you can adjust the amount of milk according to your preference.

Ingredients:

Freshly boiled water
Quality loose-leaf black tea (Assam, Darjeeling, or English Breakfast)
Milk (whole milk or semi-skimmed, to taste)
Sugar or honey (optional)

Directions:

1. Start by heating water in a kettle until it reaches a rolling boil.
2. The water should be freshly boiled for the best flavor.
3. Warm your teapot by swirling a little hot water inside, then pour it out.
4. Add one tsp. of loose-leaf black tea per person into the teapot.
5. Pour the boiled water over the tea leaves in the teapot.
6. Use approximately one cup (240ml) of water per person.
7. Stir the tea leaves gently.
8. Place the lid on the teapot and let the tea steep for about 3-5 minutes, depending on your preferred strength.
9. If you like a stronger brew, you can steep it for a bit longer.
10. While the tea is steeping, warm the milk in a small saucepan or microwave, but avoid boiling it.
11. After the steeping time is up, pour the brewed tea into teacups through a strainer to catch the tea leaves.
12. Add a splash of warm milk to each cup, adjusting the amount to your liking.
13. If desired, sweeten the tea with a little sugar or honey.
14. Stir gently to mix in the milk and sweetener.

Cucumber and Cream Cheese Finger Sandwiches

Ingredients:

Sliced white bread (crusts removed)
English cucumber, thinly sliced
Cream cheese
Fresh dill (optional)
Salt and pepper to taste

Directions:

1. Spread a thin layer of cream cheese on each slice of bread.
2. Arrange cucumber slices on one slice, season with salt, pepper, and dill (if using).
3. Top with another slice of bread, and gently press together.
4. Cut into fingers or triangles.

Smoked Salmon and Cream Cheese Sandwiches

Ingredients:

Sliced brown bread (crusts removed)
Smoked salmon
Cream cheese
Fresh lemon juice
Fresh dill (optional)

Directions:

1. Spread cream cheese on each slice of bread.
2. Lay smoked salmon on one slice, drizzle with lemon juice, and sprinkle some fresh dill (if using).
3. Top with another slice of bread, and gently press together.
4. Cut into fingers or rectangles.

Smoked Salmon and Dill Finger Sandwiches

Ingredients:

Smoked salmon slices
Cream cheese
Fresh dill
Lemon zest
Bread slices (rye or pumpernickel)

Directions:

1. Spread a thin layer of cream cheese on each bread slice.
2. Lay the smoked salmon over the cream cheese on one slice.
3. Sprinkle with fresh dill and a little lemon zest.
4. Top with the other bread slice, cream cheese side down.
5. Cut into finger sandwiches.

Egg Salad Finger Sandwiches

Ingredients:
Hard-boiled eggs, chopped
Mayonnaise
Dijon mustard
Chopped chives or green onions
Salt and pepper
Bread slices (white or whole wheat)

Directions:
1. In a bowl, mix the chopped hard-boiled eggs with mayonnaise, Dijon mustard, chopped chives or green onions, salt, and pepper to taste.
2. Spread the egg salad over one bread slice and cover with another bread slice.
3. Cut into finger sandwiches.

Roast Beef and Horseradish Finger Sandwiches

Ingredients:

Thinly sliced roast beef
Horseradish sauce
Arugula or watercress leaves
Bread slices (white or whole wheat)

Directions:

1. Spread a thin layer of horseradish sauce on each bread slice.
2. Lay the roast beef slices over the sauce on one slice.
3. Top with arugula or watercress leaves, and then place the other bread slice on top.
4. Trim the crusts and cut into finger sandwiches.

Pesto and Tomato Finger Sandwiches

Ingredients:

Basil pesto
Sliced tomatoes
Fresh mozzarella cheese
Bread slices (white or whole wheat)

Directions:

1. Spread a layer of basil pesto on one side of each bread slice.
2. Lay the sliced tomatoes and fresh mozzarella cheese over the pesto on one slice.
3. Top with the other bread slice, pesto side down.
4. Cut into finger sandwiches.

Classic British Scones

Light, fluffy baked goods often served with clotted cream and jam.

Ingredients:

2 1/2 cups all-purpose flour
2 tsps. baking powder
1/2 tsp. salt
1/4 cup unsalted butter, cold and cubed
3 tbsps. granulated sugar
2/3 cup milk
1 tsp. vanilla extract
1 egg, beaten (for egg wash)
Clotted cream and strawberry jam, to serve

Directions:

1. Preheat your oven to 400°F (200°C) and line a baking sheet with parchment paper.
2. In a large bowl, whisk together the flour, baking powder, and salt.
3. Add the cold cubed butter and rub it into the flour mixture with your fingertips until it resembles fine breadcrumbs.
4. Stir in the sugar, then add the milk and vanilla extract.
5. Mix until it forms a soft dough.
6. Turn the dough out onto a floured surface and gently knead it a few times. Roll out the dough to about 1-inch (2.5cm) thickness.
7. Use a round cookie cutter (about 2 inches/5cm in diameter) to cut out scones. Place them on the prepared baking sheet.
8. Brush the tops of the scones with the beaten egg for a golden finish.
9. Bake in the preheated oven for 12-15 minutes or until the scones are golden brown and cooked through.
10. Let the scones cool slightly before serving.

11. Serve with clotted cream and strawberry jam.

Fruit Scones

Ingredients:
2 cups all-purpose flour
1/4 cup granulated sugar
1 tbsp. baking powder
1/2 tsp. salt
1/2 cup unsalted butter, cold and cubed
2/3 cup milk
1 large egg, beaten (for egg wash)
1/2 cup dried fruit (such as raisins, currants, or sultanas)

Directions:
1. Preheat your oven to 400°F (200°C).
2. Line a baking sheet with parchment paper.
3. In a large mixing bowl, whisk together the all-purpose flour, granulated sugar, baking powder, and salt.
4. Add the cold, cubed butter to the dry ingredients.
5. Use your fingertips or a pastry cutter to rub the butter into the flour mixture until it resembles coarse crumbs.
6. Make a well in the center of the mixture and pour in the milk.
7. Mix until the dough comes together.
8. Turn the dough out onto a lightly floured surface and gently knead it a few times to make it smooth.
9. Roll out the dough to about 1-inch (2.5cm) thickness. Sprinkle the dried fruit over the dough.
10. Fold the dough over the fruit and gently knead it a few more times to distribute the fruit evenly.
11. Roll out the dough again to about 1-inch thickness. Use a floured round cookie cutter (about 2 inches or 5cm in diameter) to cut out scones.
12. Place the scones on the prepared baking sheet, leaving some space between each.
13. Brush the tops of the scones with beaten egg for a golden finish.
14. Bake the scones in the preheated oven for about 12-15 minutes or until they are lightly golden.

15. Remove from the oven and let them cool on a wire rack.
16. Serve with clotted cream and jam.

Cheese Scones

Ingredients:

2 cups all-purpose flour
1 tbsp. baking powder
1/2 tsp. salt
1/4 tsp. cayenne pepper (optional)
1/2 cup unsalted butter, cold and cubed
1 cup grated cheddar cheese
2/3 cup milk
1 large egg, beaten (for egg wash)

Directions:

1. Preheat your oven to 400°F (200°C). Line a baking sheet with parchment paper.
2. In a large mixing bowl, whisk together the all-purpose flour, baking powder, salt, and cayenne pepper (if using).
3. Add the cold, cubed unsalted butter to the dry ingredients. Use your fingertips or a pastry cutter to rub the butter into the flour mixture until it resembles coarse crumbs.
4. Stir in the grated cheddar cheese.
5. Make a well in the center of the mixture and pour in the milk.
6. Mix until the dough comes together.
7. Turn the dough out onto a lightly floured surface and gently knead it a few times to make it smooth.
8. Roll out the dough to about 1-inch (2.5cm) thickness. Use a floured round cookie cutter (about 2 inches or 5cm in diameter) to cut out scones.
9. Place the scones on the prepared baking sheet, leaving some space between each.
10. Brush the tops of the scones with beaten egg for a golden finish.
11. Bake the scones in the preheated oven for about 12-15 minutes or until they are lightly golden.
12. Remove the scones from the oven and let them cool on a wire rack. Serve with clotted cream and jam.

Sweet Pastries and Cakes

British sweet pastries and cakes form a symphony of delectable delights that have become an integral part of the country's culinary fabric. With a history dating back centuries, these sweet treats have evolved into an irresistible fusion of traditional recipes and modern innovations, capturing the essence of British baking.

Step into a charming tearoom, and you'll be greeted by the inviting aroma of freshly baked scones, adorned with clotted cream and luscious fruit preserves.
The timeless elegance of Victoria Sponge Cake beckons with its delicate layers of sponge, filled with a sweet harmony of jam and cream.

Venture deeper into this world of sweetness, and you'll discover the beloved Bakewell Tart, an enchanting blend of almond frangipane and tangy jam, encased in a crisp pastry shell. Meanwhile, Sticky Toffee Pudding entices with its moist and rich texture, steeped in a sumptuous toffee sauce.

Eton Mess dances on the palate, a playful medley of crushed meringue, velvety whipped cream, and fresh berries, offering a delightful balance of flavors and textures.

These sweet creations have found their way into homes and hearts, woven into festive celebrations, afternoon tea gatherings, and everyday indulgences. British sweet pastries and cakes are not merely desserts; they are cherished traditions that bring people together, creating moments of joy and nostalgia.

With each delectable bite, you embark on a journey through time, savoring the artistry and passion of British bakers who continue to add new layers of creativity to these time-honored delights.

From the charming countryside tearoom to the bustling city bakery, British sweet pastries and cakes stand as a testament to the rich tapestry of flavors and traditions that define the nation's love affair with all things sweet. As you savor each mouthful, you'll be reminded of the warmth and camaraderie that surrounds these beloved treats, making them an integral part of British culinary heritage for generations to come.

Mini Victoria Sponge Cakes

Ingredients:

7/8 cup unsalted butter, softened (about 14 tbsps.)
1 cup + 2 tbsps. granulated sugar
4 large eggs
1 3/4 cups self-raising flour
1 tsp. baking powder
1 tsp. vanilla extract
Strawberry jam
Whipped cream

Directions:

1. Preheat your oven to 350°F (180°C) and line a muffin tin with cupcake liners.
2. In a large bowl, beat the softened butter and sugar together until light and fluffy.
3. Beat in the eggs, one at a time, and add the vanilla extract.
4. Sift in the self-raising flour and baking powder, then gently fold the mixture until just combined.
5. Spoon the batter into the cupcake liners, filling each about two-thirds full.
6. Bake for approximately 15-18 minutes or until a toothpick inserted into the center of a cake comes out clean.
7. Let the cakes cool completely on a wire rack.
8. To assemble, slice each cake in half horizontally.
9. Spread strawberry jam on one half and top with a dollop of whipped cream.
10. Place the other half on top like a sandwich.

Crumpets

Soft, round yeast-based cakes with a characteristic honeycomb texture, typically enjoyed with butter.

Ingredients:

2 cups all-purpose flour
1 tsp. sugar
1 tsp. instant yeast
1 tsp. baking powder
1 1/4 cups warm milk
1/4 cup warm water
1/2 tsp. salt
Vegetable oil or butter for greasing

Directions:

1. In a mixing bowl, whisk together the flour, sugar, instant yeast, and baking powder until well combined.
2. Gradually pour in the warm milk and warm water while stirring the mixture to form a smooth, thick batter.
3. Add the salt to the batter and mix it in thoroughly.
4. Cover the bowl with a clean kitchen towel or plastic wrap and let the batter rest in a warm place for about 1 hour.
5. During this time, the batter should rise and become bubbly.
6. After the resting period, lightly grease a griddle or non-stick frying pan with vegetable oil or butter and place it over medium heat.
7. Using crumpet rings (or egg rings), place them onto the greased griddle or pan and pour about 1/4 cup of the batter into each ring.
8. If you don't have rings, you can simply spoon the batter directly onto the griddle, forming circular shapes.
9. Cook the crumpets over medium-low heat for about 6-8 minutes or until the surface starts to set and bubbles form on the top.

10. The crumpets should be cooked gently to ensure they cook through without burning.
11. Carefully remove the rings (if using) and flip the crumpets over using a spatula.
12. Cook the crumpets on the other side for an additional 2-3 minutes until they are golden brown.
13. Once cooked, transfer the crumpets to a wire rack to cool slightly.
14. The crumpets will have a soft, spongy texture with those characteristic holes on the top.
15. Serve the crumpets warm with a generous spread of butter and your favorite jam or honey.

British Snacks

British snacks encompass a delightful assortment of sweet and savory treats that cater to a range of tastes and preferences. Walkers Crisps, known as Lay's in other parts of the world, are one of the most popular savory snacks in the UK. With an extensive array of flavors, from classic salt and vinegar to unique options like prawn cocktail and roast chicken, Walkers Crisps offer a satisfying crunch and burst of flavor that has made them a favorite among snack enthusiasts of all ages.

On the sweet side, chocolate bars hold a special place in British snacking culture. Brands like Cadbury, Nestlé, and Mars offer an enticing selection of chocolate treats, including the iconic Cadbury Dairy Milk, Flake, and Twix bars. Jaffa Cakes, a unique combination of sponge cake, orange jelly, and chocolate, are a beloved biscuit (cookie) that straddles the line between snack and dessert. Another popular sweet snack is the beloved scone, often served with clotted cream and jam as part of a traditional afternoon tea spread.

British snacks are not only delicious but also reflect the country's culinary heritage and diverse influences. Whether you're craving a savory delight or a sweet indulgence, British snacks offer a delectable array of options that cater to any snacker's desires. From the iconic crisps to the comforting scones, these treats are perfect for satisfying hunger pangs or enjoying a little moment of pleasure throughout the day.

Homemade Crisps (Potato Chips)

The British have a wide variety of crisps in different flavors, from the traditional salt and vinegar to more unique options like prawn cocktail and roast beef.

Ingredients:

3-4 large russet potatoes (or any other variety suitable for frying)
Vegetable oil, for frying
Salt, to taste

Optional seasonings Ingredients:

Paprika
Black pepper
Garlic powder
Onion powder, or any other preferred seasoning

Directions:

1. Wash and peel the potatoes. Using a mandoline slicer or a sharp knife, thinly slice the potatoes into uniform slices. Soak the potato slices in a bowl of cold water for about 30 minutes to remove excess starch.
2. After soaking, drain the potato slices and pat them dry with a clean kitchen towel or paper towels.
3. In a large, deep saucepan or a deep fryer, heat vegetable oil to about 350°F (175°C). Make sure there's enough oil to submerge the potato slices.
4. Fry the potato slices in batches to avoid overcrowding. Carefully add a handful of slices to the hot oil and fry for about 2-3 minutes or until they turn golden and crispy. Keep an eye on them to prevent burning.
5. Using a slotted spoon, remove the fried crisps from the oil and place them on a plate lined with paper towels to absorb any excess oil. Season the hot crisps immediately with salt and any other preferred seasonings.
6. Repeat the frying process with the remaining batches of potato slices until all the crisps are cooked.

7. Let the homemade crisps cool completely before storing them in an airtight container to maintain their crispiness.

Digestive Biscuits

Digestive biscuits are sweet, semi-sweet, or plain biscuits that are often enjoyed with a cup of tea. They have a slightly crumbly texture and are made with wholemeal flour.

Ingredients:

1 1/4 cups (150g) whole wheat flour (wholemeal flour)
1/2 cup (60g) all-purpose flour
1/2 cup (100g) granulated sugar
1 tsp. baking powder
1/4 tsp. salt
1/2 cup (115g) unsalted butter, cold and cubed
1/4 cup (60ml) milk
1 tsp. vanilla extract

Directions:

1. Preheat your oven to 350°F (180°C). Line a baking sheet with parchment paper.
2. In a large mixing bowl, whisk together the whole wheat flour, all-purpose flour, granulated sugar, baking powder, and salt.
3. Add the cold, cubed unsalted butter to the dry ingredients.
4. Use your fingers or a pastry cutter to rub the butter into the flour mixture until it resembles coarse crumbs.
5. In a separate bowl, mix the milk and vanilla extract together.
6. Gradually add the milk mixture to the flour-butter mixture, stirring until a dough forms.
7. Be careful not to overmix.
8. Turn the dough out onto a lightly floured surface and knead it gently until smooth.
9. Roll out the dough to a thickness of about 1/4 in. (6mm).
10. Using a round cookie cutter or a drinking glass, cut out the biscuits and place them on the prepared baking sheet.
11. Prick each biscuit with a fork to create the classic digestive biscuit pattern.

12. Bake the biscuits in the preheated oven for approximately 12-15 minutes or until they are lightly golden around the edges.
13. Remove the biscuits from the oven and let them cool on a wire rack.
14. Once cooled, store the digestive biscuits in an airtight container to maintain their freshness.

Scotch Eggs

Hard-boiled eggs wrapped in sausage meat, coated in breadcrumbs, and deep-fried.

Ingredients:

4 large eggs
1 pound (450g) pork sausage meat (You can use sausages with casings removed if you can't find loose sausage meat)
1/2 cup all-purpose flour
1 cup breadcrumbs (You can use store-bought or make your own by processing stale bread)
1 tsp. dried thyme or sage (optional, for extra flavor)
Salt and pepper, to taste
Vegetable oil, for frying

Directions:

1. Start by preparing the eggs. Place the eggs in a saucepan and cover them with cold water.
2. Bring the water to a boil, then reduce the heat to a gentle simmer and cook the eggs for about 7-8 minutes for a slightly soft yolk or 9-10 minutes for a fully set yolk.
3. Once the eggs are cooked, immediately transfer them to a bowl of ice water to cool and stop the cooking process.
4. Let them sit in the ice water for about 5 minutes, then peel the shells off carefully. Set aside.
5. In a bowl, combine the sausage meat with dried thyme or sage (if using), and season with salt and pepper.
6. Mix everything together until well combined.
7. Divide the sausage meat mixture into four equal portions. Flatten one portion in the palm of your hand to create a disc shape.
8. Place a peeled hard-boiled egg in the center of the sausage meat disc. Carefully mold the meat around the egg, ensuring it is evenly covered. Repeat this step for the remaining eggs.

9. Set up a breading station. Place the flour in one shallow bowl, whisk the remaining eggs in another bowl, and put the breadcrumbs in a third bowl.
10. Roll each sausage-covered egg in the flour, shaking off any excess.
11. Dip it into the beaten egg, making sure it's coated all over. Finally, roll the egg in the breadcrumbs until it's completely covered.
12. Repeat for all the eggs.
13. Heat vegetable oil in a deep saucepan or a deep fryer to about 350°F (175°C).
14. Carefully lower the Scotch eggs into the hot oil and fry them for about 5-6 minutes until they are golden brown and crispy.
15. Once cooked, remove the Scotch eggs from the oil with a slotted spoon and place them on a plate lined with paper towels to drain any excess oil.
16. Serve the Scotch eggs warm or at room temperature.
17. They are delicious on their own or with some mustard or a side salad.

Pork Pies

Individual-sized pies filled with seasoned pork and enclosed in a crispy pastry crust.

Crust Pastry Ingredients:

3 cups all-purpose flour
1 tsp. salt
1/2 cup unsalted butter
1/2 cup lard or vegetable shortening
1/2 cup water

Pork Filling Ingredients:

1 pound (450g) ground pork
1 small onion, finely chopped
1 clove garlic, minced
1 tsp. dried sage
1/2 tsp. dried thyme
1/2 tsp. ground black pepper
1/2 tsp. salt
1 pinch of cayenne pepper (optional)
1 tbsp. Worcestershire sauce
1 tbsp. tomato paste

Assembling and Glazing Ingredients:

1 egg, beaten (for egg wash)
A little milk or water (for egg wash)
1 tbsp. melted butter or vegetable oil (for brushing)

Crust Pastry Directions:

1. In a large mixing bowl, whisk together the flour and salt.
2. In a saucepan, melt the butter and lard (or vegetable shortening) with water over low heat until fully melted.
3. Pour the melted fat and water mixture into the flour mixture, stirring with a spoon until a dough forms.
4. Turn the dough out onto a lightly floured surface and knead it gently until smooth.

5. Wrap the pastry dough in plastic wrap and let it rest at room temperature for about 30 minutes.

Pork Filling Directions:

1. In a skillet or frying pan, cook the ground pork over medium heat until it's no longer pink.
2. Add the chopped onion and minced garlic to the cooked pork, and continue to cook until the onion becomes translucent.
3. Stir in the dried sage, dried thyme, black pepper, salt, and cayenne pepper (if using).
4. Add Worcestershire sauce and tomato paste, mixing well to combine.
5. Remove the skillet from the heat and let the pork filling cool slightly.

Assembling Pork Pies Directions:

1. Preheat your oven to 375°F (190°C).
2. Grease a muffin tin or individual pie molds with butter or vegetable oil.
3. Divide the hot water crust pastry into two portions: two-thirds for the base and one-third for the lid.
4. Roll out the larger portion of the pastry on a lightly floured surface to about 1/8-inch (3mm) thickness.
5. Use a round cutter or a large drinking glass to cut out circles of pastry, large enough to line the base and sides of each muffin cup.
6. Press the pastry circles gently into the muffin cups, making sure they cover the base and sides evenly.
7. Fill each pastry-lined cup with the cooled pork filling, pressing it down gently to make room for the lid.
8. Roll out the smaller portion of the pastry and cut out slightly smaller circles to use as lids for the pies.
9. Place the pastry lids on top of each pie, pressing the edges to seal them with the base.

Glazing and Baking Directions:

1. In a small bowl, mix the beaten egg with a little milk or water to create an egg wash.

2. Brush the tops of the pies with the egg wash for a golden finish.
3. Make a small hole in the center of each pie lid to allow steam to escape while baking.
4. Place the filled pies on a baking sheet and bake in the preheated oven for about 25-30 minutes or until the pastry is golden and cooked through.
5. Remove the pork pies from the oven, and while they are still hot, brush the tops with melted butter or vegetable oil for added shine and flavor.
6. Let the pork pies cool slightly before serving. They can be enjoyed warm or at room temperature.

Cornish Pasty

A pastry filled with beef, potatoes, onions, and swede (rutabaga), perfect for a hearty snack.

Ingredients:

For the Pastry:
2 1/2 cups all-purpose flour
1/2 tsp. salt
1/2 cup unsalted butter, cold and cubed
1/2 cup cold water

Filling Ingredients:

1 1/2 cups beef skirt steak or chuck, diced into small cubes
1 large potato, peeled and diced into small cubes
1 small onion, finely chopped
1 small rutabaga (swede) or turnip, peeled and diced into small cubes
Salt and pepper to taste

Assembly Ingredients:

1 egg, beaten (for egg wash)

Directions:

1. In a large mixing bowl, combine the all-purpose flour and salt.
2. Add the cold, cubed unsalted butter.
3. Using your fingertips or a pastry cutter, rub the butter into the flour until the mixture resembles fine breadcrumbs.
4. Gradually add cold water to the flour-butter mixture, a little at a time, and mix until a dough forms.
5. Be careful not to overmix.
6. Shape the dough into a ball, wrap it in plastic wrap, and refrigerate it for at least 30 minutes.
7. Preheat your oven to 400°F (200°C). Line a baking sheet with parchment paper.

8. In a separate bowl, combine the diced beef, potato, onion, and rutabaga (or turnip).
9. Season the filling mixture with salt and pepper to taste.
10. On a lightly floured surface, roll out the chilled pastry dough to a thickness of about 1/8 inch (3mm).
11. Using a plate or a pastry cutter, cut the rolled-out dough into circles of about 8 inches (20cm) in diameter.
12. Place a generous amount of the filling mixture on one half of each pastry circle, leaving a border around the edges.
13. Fold the other half of the pastry circle over the filling to form a semi-circle. Press the edges together firmly to seal.
14. Crimp the sealed edges using your fingers or a fork to create a decorative border.
15. Place the pasties on the prepared baking sheet.
16. Brush the tops with beaten egg for a golden finish.
17. Bake the Cornish Pasties in the preheated oven for about 35-40 minutes or until the pastry is golden brown and the filling is cooked through.
18. Remove the pasties from the oven and let them cool slightly before serving.

British Drinks

British drinks encompass a wide range of beverages that reflect the nation's diverse tastes and cultural influences. Tea, perhaps the most iconic British drink, holds a special place in the hearts of the British people. With a rich history dating back to the 17th century, tea is an integral part of British daily life and social gatherings. Whether it's a comforting cup of English Breakfast tea in the morning or a traditional afternoon tea spread, tea is a symbol of hospitality and British tradition.

In addition to tea, another quintessential British drink is ale and beer.
The United Kingdom boasts a vibrant brewing culture, with ales, bitters, and stouts being particularly popular. Many local pubs and breweries offer an array of unique and well-crafted beers, making the pub culture an essential aspect of British social life. Pimm's, a gin-based fruit cup, is another famous British beverage, often enjoyed during the summer months. Served over ice with various fruits and herbs, Pimm's is a refreshing and light drink that embodies the spirit of British summer gatherings and sporting events.

The British also have a strong affinity for classic spirits, with gin being a notable favorite. Gin and tonic, served with a slice of lemon or lime, is a timeless and refreshing choice for many. Furthermore, whisky (often referred to as Scotch) holds a special place in British drinking culture, with Scotland being renowned for its whisky production. Whether it's a cup of tea in the morning, a pint of ale at the local pub, or a gin and tonic in the evening, British drinks reflect the country's rich traditions, diverse tastes, and enduring love for conviviality.

British Earl Grey Tea

Ingredients:

1 teaspoon loose Earl Grey tea leaves (or 1 tea bag)
1 cup water
Milk (optional)
Sugar or sweetener (optional)
Tea infuser or tea strainer

Directions:

1. Bring water to a boil in a kettle or a saucepan.
2. Once the water is boiling, remove it from the heat and let it sit for a moment to allow the temperature to slightly cool. The ideal temperature for brewing Earl Grey Tea is around 200°F (93°C).
3. While the water is cooling, add the loose Earl Grey tea leaves to a teapot or a tea infuser placed inside a cup. Alternatively, use an Earl Grey tea bag.
4. Pour the hot water over the tea leaves in the teapot or cup.
5. Fill it to the desired level based on how strong you prefer your tea.
6. Let the tea steep for 3-4 minutes. Earl Grey tea can become bitter if oversteeped, so it's best to keep the steeping time relatively short.
7. After the steeping time, remove the tea leaves by either taking out the infuser or removing the tea bag.
8. If you prefer, you can use a tea strainer to pour the tea into a separate cup.
9. If you like your tea with milk, add a splash of milk to your taste.
10. Some people prefer to add milk before pouring the tea, while others add it afterward.
11. Sweeten your tea with sugar, honey, or your preferred sweetener, if desired.
12. Give the tea a gentle stir, and it's ready to enjoy!

Flat White Coffee

Coffee drinking has become increasingly popular in the United Kingdom over the years. While tea has historically been the more traditional and prevalent hot beverage in Britain, coffee culture has grown significantly, particularly in urban areas and among younger generations.

Coffee shops and cafes can be found in most towns and cities across the UK, offering a variety of coffee options, including espressos, cappuccinos, lattes, flat whites, and more. Many British households also have coffee makers or espresso machines, allowing people to enjoy coffee in the comfort of their homes. Flat White is a very popular British coffee choice.

Ingredients:

1-2 shots of espresso (about 2 ounces/60ml)
6 ounces (180ml) steamed milk
A thin layer of microfoam (steamed milk with tiny bubbles) on top

Directions:

1. Prepare 1-2 shots of espresso using an espresso machine.
2. In a separate milk pitcher, steam the milk until it reaches a silky and velvety texture, with a thin layer of microfoam on top.
3. The milk should be heated to around 150°F (65°C), but be careful not to overheat it, as this can scald the milk and affect the flavor.
4. Pour the steamed milk over the espresso in a slow and steady stream, aiming to create a creamy and balanced coffee drink with a smooth texture.
5. The Flat White should have a rich flavor, with the espresso and steamed milk blending harmoniously, and the microfoam providing a velvety mouthfeel.
6. Optionally, you can add a sprinkle of cocoa or cinnamon on top for a touch of additional flavor.

Pimm's Cup

A refreshing summer cocktail made with Pimm's No. 1, lemonade, and various fruits and herbs.

Ingredients:

2 oz (60ml) Pimm's No. 1
3-4 oz (90-120ml) lemonade or lemon-lime soda (e.g., Sprite or 7-Up)
Ice cubes
Fresh fruits (such as strawberries, cucumber slices, orange slices, and mint leaves)
Optional garnish: A sprig of fresh mint and a slice of lemon or cucumber

Directions:

1. Fill a tall glass with ice cubes.
2. Add the fresh fruits into the glass. You can use a combination of strawberries, cucumber slices, orange slices, and mint leaves. This is a great opportunity to get creative and use seasonal fruits you have on hand.
3. Pour the Pimm's No. 1 over the ice and fruits in the glass.
4. Top up the glass with lemonade or lemon-lime soda. You can adjust the amount of lemonade based on your desired sweetness.
5. Give the cocktail a gentle stir to combine the ingredients and distribute the flavors.
6. If desired, garnish the Pimm's Cup with a sprig of fresh mint and a slice of lemon or cucumber.
7. Serve immediately and enjoy your refreshing Pimm's Cup!
8. Note: Pimm's Cup is a versatile cocktail, and you can adjust the ingredients to suit your taste. Some people like to add a splash of ginger ale or lemonade for extra sweetness.

9. Additionally, you can create a large pitcher of Pimm's Cup for a group gathering by increasing the quantities of each ingredient and adjusting to taste.

Mulled Wine

A warm, spiced wine often enjoyed during the festive season.

Ingredients:

1 bottle (750ml) red wine (use a medium-bodied red wine like Merlot, Cabernet Sauvignon, or Shiraz)
1/4 cup brandy or rum (optional, for an extra kick)
1/4 cup honey or sugar (adjust to taste)
1 orange, sliced
8-10 whole cloves
2 cinnamon sticks
2-3 star anise
1-2 whole allspice berries (optional)
1-2 cardamom pods (optional)
Additional orange slices, cinnamon sticks, and star anise for garnish (optional)

Directions:

1. Pour the red wine into a large saucepan or a slow cooker.
2. Add the brandy or rum (if using) to the wine.
3. Stir in the honey or sugar until it's fully dissolved.
4. Adjust the sweetness to your preference.
5. Add the orange slices to the wine mixture.
6. Stud the orange slices with the whole cloves, pushing the cloves into the orange peel.
7. Add the cinnamon sticks, star anise, and any other optional spices you prefer, like allspice berries or cardamom pods.
8. Gently heat the mixture over low to medium heat (or use the "low" setting on a slow cooker).
9. Be careful not to let it boil as you want to retain the alcohol content.
10. Let the mulled wine simmer for about 15-20 minutes, allowing the flavors to infuse into the wine.
11. Stir occasionally to ensure the flavors are well distributed.

12. Taste the mulled wine and adjust the sweetness or spiciness if necessary. You can add more honey/sugar for sweetness or more spices if you want a stronger flavor.
13. Once the mulled wine is heated through and well infused, it's ready to serve.
14. Ladle the mulled wine into mugs or heatproof glasses, making sure to include some of the fruits and spices in each serving.
15. Optionally, garnish with additional orange slices, cinnamon sticks, or star anise for a festive touch.
16. Serve the mulled wine warm and enjoy the cozy and comforting flavors!

About the Author

Laura Sommers is **The Recipe Lady!**

She lives on a small farm in Baltimore County, Maryland and has a passion for food. She has taken cooking classes in New York City, Memphis, New Orleans and Washington DC. She has been a taste tester for a large spice company in Baltimore and written food reviews for several local papers. She loves writing cookbooks with the most delicious recipes to share her knowledge and love of cooking with the world.

Follow her on Pinterest:

http://pinterest.com/therecipelady1

Visit the Recipe Lady's blog for even more great recipes:

http://the-recipe-lady.blogspot.com/

Visit her Amazon Author Page to see her latest books:

amazon.com/author/laurasommers

Follow the Recipe Lady on Facebook:

https://www.facebook.com/therecipegirl

Follow her on Twitter:

https://twitter.com/TheRecipeLady1

Other Books by Laura Sommers

Irish Recipes for St. Patrick's Day

Traditional Vermont Recipes

Traditional Memphis Recipes

Maryland Chesapeake Bay Blue Crab Cookbook

Mussels Cookbook

Maryland Chesapeake Bay Blue Crab Cookbook

Salmon Cookbook

Scallop Recipes

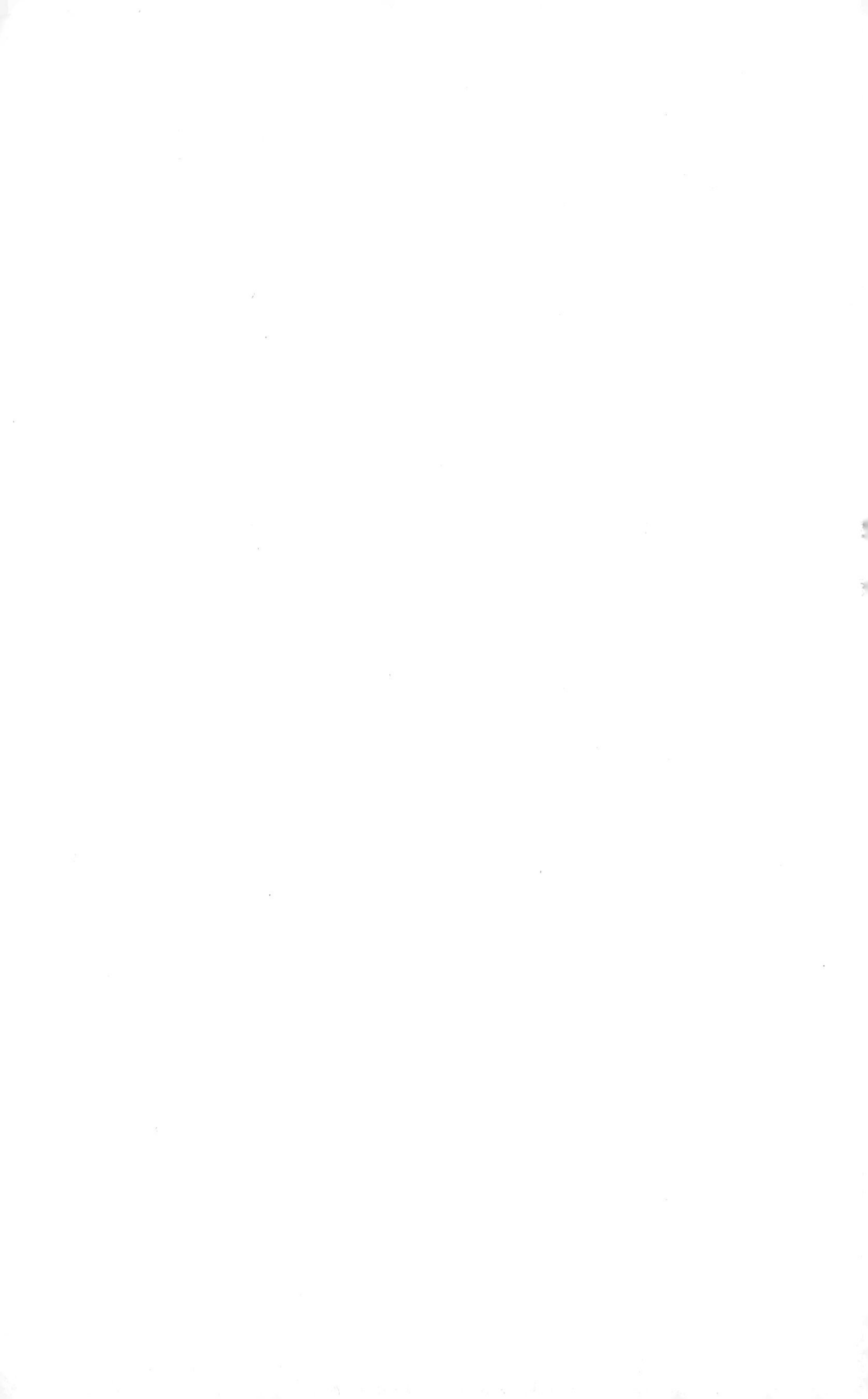

Made in the USA
Columbia, SC
11 December 2024

Copyright © 2024 by Gleanit Books

ALL RIGHTS RESERVED. No part of this book may be reproduced or transmitted in any form by any means, electronic or mechanical, including photocopying and recording, or by any information storage and retrieval system, except as may be expressly permitted in writing by the Author.

The information in this book related to exercise, fitness, diet, and nutrition is intended for informational purposes only. You should consult with a physician before beginning any lifestyle transformation routine. Nothing contained in this book should be considered medical advice or diagnosis. The Publisher and Author assume no responsibility for errors and omissions. Neither is any liability assumed for damages resulting from the use of information contained herein.

A MEAL A DAY–A LIFESTYLE BEYOND NUTRITION AND FITNESS

By OMO OIBOH

*To my kids Elora, Brisa, and James and the readers of this book.
All you desire is already within you!*

CONTENTS

INTRODUCTION 1
1. THE BASICS OF OMAD 6
2. GROWTH MINDSET: IMPLEMENTING INCREMENTAL CHANGES 18
3. BALANCED NUTRIENT-DENSE DIET 31
4. INTEGRATING EXERCISE 56
5. BALANCING OMAD DIET AND EXERCISE 77
6. OVERCOMING CHALLENGES 83
7. DOCUMENTING THE JOURNEY 96
8. EMPOWERING WELLNESS 122
9. GETTING STARTED 127
CONCLUSION 142
APPENDIX 144
NOTES 145
GLOSSARY 155
INDEX 158

INTRODUCTION

I invite my readers to join me on a journey towards a transformative lifestyle choice that has significantly enhanced my health, sharpened my mental clarity, and increased my physical vitality—the one-meal-a-day (OMAD) lifestyle. My path to this lifestyle began in January 2014, not abruptly or deliberately, but as a natural progression from my early experiments with intermittent fasting.

Before fully embracing a one-meal-a-day routine, I noticed that altering my eating patterns—such as having only coffee in the morning and delaying my meal to later in the day—had surprisingly positive effects. It helped me stay more focused during work, and I felt an overall improvement in my health and vitality. Conversely, having a large meal early in the day seemed to diminish my focus and negatively affect my productivity. These observations prompted me to think more critically about the relationship between my diet, physical condition, and mental state.

At this point, it's also pertinent to share that before embracing this lifestyle, I experienced challenges with maintaining a consistent weight. My weight fluctuated significantly due to inconsistency in maintaining an active lifestyle. There were periods of weight gain followed by periods of weight loss, highlighting a cycle of challenges that stemmed from a lack of dietary and lifestyle consistency. This realization highlighted the need for a more stable and practical approach to my health and well-being.

Encouraged by the initial positive impacts of intermittent fasting, I felt motivated to take things a step further by restricting myself to just one meal a day. Imagine convincing your stomach that one hearty meal is all it gets in a day. Seems daunting at first, right? Nonetheless, I was committed to the challenge, focusing on the tangible benefits I had started to notice by delaying meals. It was both a challenge and an opportunity to redefine my relationship with food and nutrition. My decision wasn't about following a diet trend but a thoughtful exploration of how this eating pattern could enhance my life.

Through this book, "A Meal a Day, A Lifestyle Beyond Nutrition and Fitness," I will share the insights and knowledge I've gained from nearly a decade of living the one-meal-a-day (OMAD) lifestyle. I aim to guide you through this life-changing journey by drawing from my own experience. The one-meal-a-day approach has been sustainable and vital in enhancing my well-being. However, it's crucial to understand that while this book leverages scientific research, my narrative offers a real-world application of these principles. This is not a substitute for medical advice but rather an addition to the existing body of knowledge, demonstrating the practical implementation of a lifestyle that has worked remarkably for me.

This book is more than just eating once a day. It represents a holistic approach to health that integrates mindful eating—

selecting a balanced, nutrient-dense meal and being conscious and present while you eat, focusing on how the food makes you feel—the strategic use of fasting to achieve optimal well-being, and a dedication to exercise, with a special focus on running, particularly half marathons. There's a specific reason why I highlight half marathons, and I'll delve into why they hold special significance for me later in the book.

My transformative journey began with running as a fundamental part of my exercise regimen, which soon became a cornerstone of my fitness routine, eventually leading me to marathon participation. By exploring different distances, I found half marathons to be the most rewarding for my physical and mental health. My exploration didn't end with running. In 2021, I expanded my athletic endeavors to include triathlons, starting with a sprint triathlon, a format known for its shorter distances. Incorporating cycling and swimming into my regimen broadened my training and significantly improved my overall fitness and stamina. Participating in these diverse athletic events deepened my appreciation for what the body can accomplish with focused dedication and an intelligent approach to nutrition and exercise.

I invite you to join me on this journey to discover the significant impact this lifestyle can have on your overall health and how it can transform your relationship with food. This book aims to clarify the OMAD lifestyle, offering a well-rounded view of its benefits and challenges and illustrating how it can be a catalyst for achieving greater health and vitality.

At its core, this narrative is a journey through the scientific, nutritional, and psychological aspects of adopting this lifestyle. However, it is more than just a diet book about the simple dichotomy of consuming and refraining from certain foods. It aims to be a companion on your journey towards a more mindful way of living, filled with actionable advice, personal stories, and the motivational lessons I've learned along the way.

Thus, this book serves as an insightful guide for those intrigued by the potential of redefining their dietary habits for better health outcomes. It offers a structured approach to understanding how a singular daily meal, when properly composed, can support rigorous physical activities, including the demanding preparation for and completion of half marathons.

For readers curious about the practicality of maintaining an active lifestyle with a minimalist dietary approach, my narrative provides both inspiration and insights. It offers practical advice and thoughts I would share with my past self if I had to begin this journey, showcasing the achievable balance between dietary restraint, nutritional adequacy, and high-level physical performance.

Through this book, I invite both men and women, from young adults to seniors, to delve into a lifestyle that combines nutrient-dense, well-balanced meals, strategic fasting, and engaging in physical activities as pillars of health and vitality. Whether you are already active in your local running community or are considering taking up running, strength training, or other exercise routines as a part of this transformative journey, the insights provided aim to inspire and steer you toward embracing the full spectrum of benefits this comprehensive approach to living offers.

The goal is to encourage adult readers globally to explore this lifestyle for themselves and to experience firsthand its significant impact on one's health, focus, and overall performance. It is about making this lifestyle accessible and achievable, regardless of one's geographical location or fitness background, and showing how it can be adapted to suit the needs and goals of adults willing to give it a try.

For younger readers, this book serves as an educational tool, offering insights into making thoughtful food choices. Although the OMAD lifestyle is not recommended for all ages, and my own journey did not start until my 30s, understanding the importance of nutrient-dense, well-balanced meals is invaluable.

So, if you've ever wondered whether you could live off one meal a day and still engage in endurance activities like marathons, precisely half marathons, as I do, you're about to find out on these pages.

Let's embark on this journey together and discover the potential for a more conscious, healthful, and fulfilling way of living. "A Meal a Day: A Lifestyle Beyond Nutrition and Fitness" is not just a book; it's a steppingstone to a wellness revolution.

1
THE BASICS OF OMAD

As we embark on the first chapter, I invite you to open your mind to a practice that might initially seem daunting—eating just once a day. However, before discussing this concept, it's essential to understand the journey that led me to its adoption.

My experience with fluctuating weight was not the catalyst for my exploration into this lifestyle. Instead, I was encouraged by the potential benefits I witnessed, such as enhanced mental clarity and focus, due to delaying meals. In my 20s, I got to work alongside seasoned experts on significant energy projects, which demanded me to be sharply focused and highly attentive. I discovered that delaying meals improved my concentration and engagement levels, enabling me to recall information much quicker and visualize abstract concepts.

Over time, as I transitioned from indiscriminate eating habits to more deliberate meal timing, I noticed both mental and physical benefits. Still, my weight fluctuated. Later, around 2017, I incorporated exercise into my routine. That's when my weight stabilized, and I started paying attention to the nutritional value of my meals. These "little wins" on the scale and beyond it, as I came to see them, were early indicators of the deep impact that meal timing and composition could have on my life. This journey of discovery laid the groundwork for the one-meal-a-day lifestyle that I would ultimately embrace.

You may ask why one would choose to eat only one meal a day. The reasons are manifold, grounded in both my personal experiences and scientific understanding. This lifestyle is not merely about reducing your calorie intake; it's about understanding your body's relationship with food, enhancing your mental clarity, and pushing your physical capabilities to new heights. My personal journey involves daily workouts, running half marathons, cycling, and participating in triathlons. It's about challenging the misconceptions surrounding fasting and demonstrating that it's possible to maintain an active, marathon-running lifestyle while embracing the discipline of consuming just one meal daily.

Adopting the one-meal-a-day lifestyle does indeed involve an initial period of adjustment. The shift from multiple meals to a single, nutritious meal may challenge your established notions of nutrition and hunger management. However, this adaptation period is a gateway to a truly transformative lifestyle. Over time, your body learns to efficiently utilize stored fats for energy, which can diminish hunger sensations and aid in managing your weight effectively, all without compromising your overall health.

The experiences of many, including my own, affirm that adopting this lifestyle can significantly boost mental and physical efficiency. Herein lies the secret to effectively adopting this method: the quality and completeness of your daily meal. It should be a meal that satiates, nourishes, and fulfills your daily nutritional needs.

While the timing of this meal can vary according to personal preference, concluding the day with this meal works best. It avoids the lethargy often associated with heavy midday meals and aligns with the body's natural rhythms, allowing for better digestion and utilization of nutrients overnight.

In the pages that follow, the concept of a meal a day will be discussed, its historical background, the theory behind this dietary lifestyle, the scientific evidence supporting it, and its profound benefits. Together, we will explore how a single meal a day, combined with an active lifestyle, can lead to unparalleled health benefits and a deeper connection with your body's needs and capabilities.

UNDERSTANDING ONE MEAL A DAY

Embracing the one-meal-a-day (OMAD) lifestyle is a progression from the broader concept of intermittent fasting or time-restricted eating, taking it to a more focused and dedicated level. Typically, intermittent fasting involves consuming your meals within a set window of 8 hours, such as from 12 pm to 8 pm, and then fasting for the remaining 16 hours of the day, sleep time included. This method is commonly known as the 16:8 fast.

However, OMAD narrows this eating window even further, resulting in a longer fasting period. However, my approach to a meal a day involves three adaptable strategies. I want readers to understand that the process is more nuanced than merely confining meals to a specific window. It's about understanding and listening to your body's needs and applying a methodical and research-backed approach to nutrition and wellness.

The routine starts each day with a focus on hydration, emphasizing the importance of drinking water right after waking up to jumpstart metabolism and prepare the body for the day ahead. Following this, I engage in a light exercise, such as a brief, low-intensity walk lasting no more than 20 minutes. Post-exercise, I would take coffee and proceed with my day's activities. The beginning of my eating window is the time when my workday finishes. This period extends to about 8 pm, during which I consume one big meal comprising a balanced mix of proteins, carbohydrates, fats, water, fruits, and vegetables. Following this main meal, I allow myself to snack if desired and stop an hour before bedtime. I followed this routine Monday to Friday. The next day, I would wake up feeling energetic from the previous meal.

In exploring variations, my second approach involved delaying my main meal to as late as 6 pm while maintaining the principle of stopping snacking an hour before sleep. This slight modification demonstrated that flexibility within an OMAD framework could still support high energy levels and sharp focus during the workweek.

The third variation introduced a more rigorous morning routine incorporating various exercises, including walking, biking, and strength training, totaling about an hour. On days when my body signaled for nourishment midday, I would opt for a light snack, such as fruit, before having my significant meal around 6 pm. This adjustment allowed for a responsive approach to my body's needs while adhering to the OMAD principle during the weekdays.

On weekends, I introduced an interesting dynamic to my OMAD journey. With a surge of energy in the mornings, attributed to the previous day's nutrition, I engaged in extended exercise sessions, sometimes lasting up to three hours. Post-exercise, I'd have my significant meal earlier, around 11am, followed by snacks as needed, based on healthy choices throughout the day. This flexibility on Saturdays and Sundays provided a refreshing break from the more structured weekday routine, contributing to a balanced and sustainable lifestyle. That was my approach to a meal a day.

As for the optimal time to have this single meal, many people practicing OMAD prefer the evening. However, there doesn't seem to be a consensus or scientific backing for this preference. The time to take your sole meal depends more on your intuition when you find it convenient and feel best.

The one-meal-a-day diet, while gaining popularity in modern wellness circles, traces its roots back through various cultures and historical periods, embodying simplicity and discipline often lost in today's fast-paced lifestyle. This resurgence in modern wellness practices brings a wealth of anecdotal and scientific support for its benefits.

Fasting, an intrinsic human behavior as natural as eating, has been part of my journey for almost a decade now. My initial encounters with intermittent fasting introduced me to its significant health benefits, notably achieving mental clarity and increased focus, which led me toward my journey of eating a meal a day.

However, even if one understands these advantages, one may harbor reservations due to disliking feeling hungry, which accompanies fasting. My goal is to address and alleviate these concerns through my personal experience, as I discovered the challenge lies not in the length of the fast but in overcoming habitual eating patterns, like evening snacks or morning sweeteners.

This adjustment phase is crucial and entirely manageable with the right mindset and strategies. Adapting to this lifestyle meant reevaluating my relationship with food, recognizing the difference between actual hunger and mere habit, and gradually shifting towards more mindful eating practices. This process helped me comfortably settle into the OMAD routine and enhanced my overall well-being, proving that with patience and diligence, one can redefine one's eating habits for the better.

Adjusting to the fasting regimen, I realized that I felt hungry because my body was accustomed to frequent meals and was unfamiliar with prolonged fasting intervals. But my journey was marked by a conscious decision to delay my meals. I was motivated by the knowledge that this self-discipline would bring significant rewards. Among these benefits, the most noticeable were a sharper mental clarity and an enhanced capacity to understand complex, abstract ideas—an invaluable asset in my field where I engaged with complex, global-scale projects. This mental strength and the noticeable improvements in concentration and alertness became vital in my successful transition to a new meal schedule.

Many individuals interested in health and wellness are keen on adopting a diet that is as similar as possible to the diet humans have followed throughout evolution. The theory is, of course, that many of our current health problems are the result of our modern diet, and if we were to eat a "Paleolithic" or primal diet, our health problems would resolve themselves.

A primal diet, incorporating periods of fasting, mirrors the historical human experience where fasting was a norm, facilitating detoxification, cell recycling, insulin reduction, and fat utilization. The constant availability of food, a relatively modern development, contrasts sharply with the human body's evolutionary design for fasting. The constant consumption that characterizes our modern eating habits deviates significantly from what is historically natural for humans.

Even with the advent of agriculture, which significantly increased food availability and reduced the necessity for fasting, many cultures and religions across the globe continued to embrace fasting both for its health benefits and as a spiritual practice. This includes well-documented traditions within Greek Orthodox Christianity, Buddhism, Islam, and Hinduism and significant practices within African cultures, such as the historic Kingdom of Benin.

In Benin, fasting was recognized for its importance in both health and spiritual disciplines, emphasizing the practice's global relevance. Esteemed historical figures like Hippocrates, Plato, and Benjamin Franklin, alongside contemporary advocates like Dr. Jason Fung, have all recognized the health merits of fasting. Dr. Fung points out that until the 1970s, it was common for people to naturally fast for 12-14 hours overnight, a stark contrast to the frequent snacking seen in today's lifestyle.

This backdrop sets the stage for the one-meal-a-day (OMAD) diet, an advanced intermittent fasting protocol that recommends including only one meal per day.

What Does a Meal a Day Do to Your Body?

When we consume food, our pancreas secretes insulin, a hormone that converts food into glucose (sugar) for immediate energy use or storage as glycogen (stored sugar) or fat.

Frequent eating keeps our insulin and blood sugar levels elevated, leading to the continuous use of glucose for energy and the accumulation of excess energy as glycogen or fat without burning any stored fat.

For the body to utilize stored fat, our insulin levels need to decrease, which occurs after a period without eating. Our body's glycogen reserves last approximately 24-36 hours, then shift to using stored fat for energy.

This principle underpins the popular "Keto diet," where the body enters a state of ketosis after one to two days of fasting. In ketosis, diminished insulin levels prompt the body to break down fat into fatty acids for energy. These fatty acids are then converted into ketone bodies, providing energy, especially for the brain.

The scientific foundation of eating one meal a day highlights significant improvements in metabolic health and a shift towards more efficient energy usage by the body. Research indicates that such dietary patterns can enhance blood sugar levels, reduce inflammation, and support weight management. For instance, a study published in the journal Cell Metabolism found intermittent fasting, closely related to OMAD, improved various health markers in participants, including reductions in body weight, blood pressure, and inflammatory markers.

Although adjusting to a new eating schedule and ensuring nutritional completeness pose challenges, they are attainable with careful planning and consideration. Also, the initial positive outcomes motivate you to believe in the process and continue the efforts. I can say this from my firsthand experience. Incorporating a diverse range of foods into a daily meal can help meet nutritional needs, while the practice encourages a mindful relationship with food, emphasizing quality over quantity. In my decade-long experience, the emphasis on choosing a diverse range of nutrient-dense foods for my daily meal was key to my approach. Quality over quantity became my mantra, focusing on vegetables, lean proteins, and healthy fats to fuel my body.

My dietary journey has been a process of evolution and discovery, beginning with intermittent fasting, transitioning into a vegetarian diet, and including a six-month hiatus from coffee. This period of abstention from coffee was enriched by the addition of herbs and herbal teas like mint, turmeric, and ginger, introducing a spectrum of health benefits and natural energy sources into my diet. These changes nourished my body and synergized with my active lifestyle and marathon training, providing the vital nutrients needed to sustain my energy levels and enhance my overall well-being.

As my dietary practices evolved, I reintegrated lean proteins and resumed coffee consumption, now complemented by the herbal teas that had become a staple in my regimen. This holistic approach underscored the versatility and adaptability of a one-meal-a-day lifestyle, proving it a robust foundation for supporting rigorous physical activity and continuous health improvement.

In embracing one meal a day, individuals embark on a journey that transcends mere dietary change into a holistic redefinition of health and well-being. This approach encourages a deeper introspection into the quantity and quality of food consumed, fostering a mindful and intentional relationship with food. It becomes a pathway to discovering how disciplined eating patterns can significantly impact physical health, mental clarity, and emotional balance, offering a comprehensive enhancement of life's quality. This lifestyle shift, rooted in my decade-long experience, has consistently demonstrated improvements in well-being, supported by a thoughtful selection of foods and a commitment to physical activity, including marathon running.

BENEFITS OF A MEAL A DAY

Physical Health Improvements

Adopting a one-meal-a-day (OMAD) lifestyle presents a myriad of benefits for physical health, including effective weight management, enhanced metabolic health, and potentially increased longevity. This lifestyle simplifies eating habits, cutting down on incessant snacking and accumulating excess calories, thus facilitating a natural reduction in body weight.

The intermittent fasting component inherent in OMAD lowers insulin levels, shifting the body's energy source from glucose to stored fat, thereby promoting fat loss without compromising nutritional health.

Moreover, athletes and individuals engaged in sports training may find that OMAD enhances their body's efficiency in fat burning. Experts explain that engaging in physical activity while in a fasted state enhances the muscle's ability to utilize fat as energy by increasing the proteins involved in fat metabolism. My experience during various athletic events, including half marathons and sprint triathlons, is a practical example of this. Competing in these demanding events without consuming food beforehand, I relied on the energy from meals consumed the previous day. This approach effectively demonstrated my body's adaptation to utilizing stored fat or energy reserves, allowing me to complete these races successfully. This capability emphasizes the body's remarkable ability to adjust to fat-burning for energy, especially during prolonged physical activities, without the immediate need for food intake before the event. This adaptation aids in overcoming the common challenge of "hitting the wall" and supports endurance and performance.

From my personal experience with this lifestyle, the clear and significant benefits to health are unmistakable. Remarkably, I have had no need to visit a doctor for any health-related issues, nor have I experienced even minor ailments like headaches. Throughout this period, including during the pandemic, my health remained robust without needing medications such as Tylenol. This was further confirmed when, at age 40, a comprehensive health check-up revealed optimal health indicators. This experience highlights the potential of OMAD to improve daily well-being and significantly reduce healthcare dependence.

Delaying meals during the day sets off various beneficial processes in our bodies. It's about engaging our bodies to promote better health and well-being, from improved metabolic health to a clearer mind. By adopting this practice, I did not just change when to eat but enhanced how my body operates, leading to noticeable improvements in my physical and mental health.

Evidence says that delaying meals during the day boosts adrenaline levels, enhancing our metabolism and energy levels. Human Growth Hormone (HGH) production also rises, aiding muscle preservation and decelerating the aging process.

Additionally, fasting boosts the generation of brain-derived neurotrophic factor (BDNF), encouraging the formation of new brain cells and connections and potentially slowing the progression of neurological conditions such as Alzheimer's, Parkinson's, and Huntington's diseases.

Another significant process induced by fasting is autophagy. This concept caught my interest and led to the 2016 Nobel Prize in Physiology or Medicine for Yoshinori Ohsumi for his autophagy discoveries. Autophagy is the body's mechanism of recycling damaged or diseased cells by breaking them down and reusing their components, leading to the creation of new, healthy cells. This process extends to the immune system, where old, damaged white blood cells are replaced with new ones upon resuming eating, effectively rejuvenating the immune system. However, autophagy is halted by high glucose, insulin, and protein levels, thus not occurring with constant eating.

Mental Clarity and Emotional Well-being

The one-meal-a-day diet notably enhances mental clarity and emotional well-being, a phenomenon supported by anecdotal accounts and scientific research. The stabilization of insulin levels plays a critical role in this process. By avoiding the frequent spikes and crashes in blood sugar associated with multiple daily meals, individuals can experience more stable energy levels and mood throughout the day, contributing to sharper focus and increased productivity.

Research Support

The benefits of the one-meal-a-day lifestyle, both physiological and psychological, are robustly supported by scientific research.

Studies have consistently demonstrated that the various health improvements associated with OMAD—from enhanced metabolic functions to increased mental clarity—are not merely anecdotal but are grounded in scientific evidence.

Research highlights the significant impact of intermittent fasting on improving insulin sensitivity, reducing inflammation, and bolstering cardiovascular health. Moreover, the neurological advantages, such as better cognitive function and mood stabilization, are linked to the hormonal and metabolic changes induced by fasting. These findings are supported by a wealth of academic papers and expert analyses, validating the comprehensive health benefits of adopting a disciplined eating pattern like OMAD.

This body of research provides a strong foundation for understanding how a simplified eating schedule can significantly improve health and well-being, making it a viable option for those seeking a scientifically backed approach to enhance their quality of life.

2

GROWTH MINDSET: IMPLEMENTING INCREMENTAL CHANGES

Initiating significant lifestyle changes stems from a realization that improvement is necessary—not just for enhancing health, appearance, or performance, but for overall well-being. This shift, however, is not instantaneous and involves more than adjusting meal frequencies. It's a comprehensive transformation that begins with a fundamental change in mindset—it demands a holistic reevaluation of our relationship with food and nutrition.

Understanding this, preparing for the OMAD lifestyle is not merely about altering meal timings; it involves a mental recalibration and a readiness to embrace new habits that align with our deeper health and wellness goals. It's about laying a solid foundation that supports the logistical aspects of OMAD and addresses the psychological and emotional willingness for a significant lifestyle shift.

Quickly transforming daily routines can be challenging. Goals such as losing weight, increasing fitness, or adopting healthier eating habits often appear as New Year's resolutions but tend to fade without a solid foundation. Therefore, recognizing the need for change is the first step toward embracing a new mindset that supports sustainable transformation.

In this chapter, I will share the steps I took to prepare for change, focusing on the essential mindset shift, cultivating patience and persistence, and setting achievable health and fitness goals. This preparation phase is crucial, as it sets the stage for a successful and sustainable transformation, ensuring that the journey to OMAD is not just about a new eating schedule but thriving within it and reaping the extensive benefits it offers.

MENTAL PREPARATION

Embarking on the OMAD journey starts with a crucial phase: Mental Preparation. This step is about understanding and integrating new, healthier habits into our lives. Research shows a large part of our day is governed by habits—automatic behaviors that play a significant role in our overall lifestyle. Recognizing and reshaping these habits is the foundation of any lasting change.

However, establishing new healthy habits (and discarding old, unhealthy ones) necessitates groundwork. Even the best intentions can fizzle out if you lose sight of the reasons behind the behavioral change. Stay connected to the motivations that prompted your decision to embark on this journey.

Acknowledging the Need for Change is key. It's about deeply connecting with the motivations driving the switch to OMAD. Focus on the "why." What prompted your choice to enhance your health, fitness, or mental well-being? Whether it's a missed opportunity that highlighted a lack of fitness, the impact of stress on your well-being, or the aspiration for sharper mental clarity at work, pinpointing these reasons strengthens your will. Any of these rationales can reinforce your dedication to change.

For me, the turning point was observing how delayed meal times significantly boosted my focus and mental performance. This wasn't just a minor improvement but a significant enhancement in how I processed information and tackled demanding tasks. I realized that spacing meals could elevate my cognitive function and overall engagement with life's tasks.

Once your mindset shifts, you're ready to face the challenges with patience and persistence. Initially, one of the primary challenges I encountered in shifting to the OMAD lifestyle was occasional hunger pangs and adjusting to a new eating schedule. Early on, I found that incorporating black coffee and sipping water throughout the day effectively curbed my appetite and maintained my focus, allowing me to stay productive.

Embracing Patience and Perseverance in Your OMAD Journey

The shift to the OMAD lifestyle is as much about mental endurance as it is about physical adaptation. From the outset, embracing patience and perseverance was crucial. Even before I had perfected my dietary choices or established a consistent exercise regimen, I began experiencing noticeable improvements in mental clarity during fasting periods. This early benefit was unexpected but encouraging, reinforcing my commitment to this lifestyle change.

The benefits multiplied as I refined my approach, integrating more nutritious foods and regular physical activity. I saw enhancements in my mental acuity, physical vitality, and endurance. This holistic improvement was motivational yet not devoid of challenges. For instance, as my participation in running events increased, so did my encounters with muscle cramps, prompting me to reassess and optimize the nutritional makeup of my daily meals.

I carefully tailored my meal composition to support my physical demands, especially on days filled with strenuous activities. I included a balanced mix of lean proteins for muscle recovery, complex carbohydrates for sustained energy, and essential fats for long-lasting satiety. Additionally, various vitamins and minerals were crucial to round out my nutritional intake, ensuring my body received all it needed to perform optimally.

This strategic nutritional planning became the cornerstone of my ability to engage in more intense and prolonged workouts. By aligning my diet closely with my physical activities, I forged a powerful synergy that allowed me to push my physical limits and enhance my overall performance. This experience highlighted the critical interplay between a well-tuned diet and physical activity, a theme that resonates throughout my journey with OMAD.

Achieving Ambitions: Preparing for the Marathon Milestone

Mental preparation and cultivating patience and persistence were foundational to my transformation. As my confidence grew alongside my energy levels, I felt encouraged to set larger, more challenging goals. The newfound vitality, particularly on weekends, inspired me to do more. This aspiration was not sudden but a result of months of dedicated training and lifestyle adjustment. It culminated in my decision to sign up for a marathon in 2019, an ambition fueled by years of watching televised events like the Houston Marathon and dreaming of participating in it.

After dedicating six months to regular, structured exercise routines, I committed to running the marathon, marking a major milestone in my lifestyle transformation. Having a whole year to prepare, I focused intensely on training, which aimed at physical preparation and reinforcing the mental and emotional resilience required for such an endeavor.

This period of preparation was not just about physical fitness; it was evidence of the mental shifts that had begun with my OMAD journey. The clear, achievable goal of completing the marathon kept me dedicated to maintaining my modified lifestyle and proved to be a powerful motivator in continuing to push the boundaries of what I thought possible.

Maintaining a Positive and Determined Mindset

I relied on several strategies and practices throughout the adjustment period to sustain a positive and determined mindset. Firstly, I recognized the efficacy of existing methods that had proven beneficial. Notably, maintaining mental clarity and incorporating nourishing foods into my diet had already yielded tangible results, and I decided to adhere to these approaches.

Setting clear objectives played a key role in maintaining my focus and motivation. My new primary target was to train for and complete a marathon. This goal provided a concrete endpoint to strive towards, serving as a driving force during challenging moments.

Consistency became a guiding principle in both my personal and professional efforts. I remained firm in my commitment to maintaining a disciplined approach to work, leveraging my interactions with skilled professionals to measure the impact of my lifestyle modifications. Observing the positive effects on both my performance and well-being backed my dedication to the journey.

Undoubtedly, it was not without its ups and downs. However, the feeling of the benefits of my efforts, transitioning from subconscious to conscious awareness, empowered me to persevere. Over time, these practices evolved into habits, and my modified lifestyle entered my daily routines.

SETTING REALISTIC GOALS

Setting Personal Health and Fitness Goals

When embarking on the one-meal-a-day lifestyle, setting personal health and fitness goals was a deliberate process guided by a desire for tangible achievements. My initial goal centered on completing a marathon—an ambitious task that required careful preparation and dedication.

I engaged in rigorous preparation and consistently put in the effort. As the marathon date approached, I incorporated a combination of walking and running into my routine and completed the 26.2 miles, ultimately crossing the finish line within the designated time frame.

However, this journey into the extremes of my physical endurance, involving activities such as running, cycling, and swimming, was not without its challenges. The challenges included muscle cramps and nutritional uncertainties that, while familiar, demanded continuous adaptation and deeper understanding. By viewing these setbacks as opportunities for further experimentation, I deepened my knowledge of how my body reacted to various physical stresses. This led to refined training and nutritional strategies, echoing the themes of learning and adaptation that were central to my holistic approach to exercise. This process was about embracing a cycle of learning and adaptation that honed my approach to both exercise and nutrition, ensuring a balanced progression across different physical activities.

Upon receiving the medal for completing the challenge, I felt great achievement. It was a powerful motivator, prompting me to seek further challenges. Building on this success, I expanded my horizons by enrolling in additional events in the same year, including participating in a half marathon in the Woodlands in the spring, followed by the Houston half marathon in the fall. Each event provided a unique opportunity for growth and strengthened my commitment to maintaining a healthy lifestyle.

The momentum gained from these achievements propelled me to set my sights on another marathon in 2020, managing to shave off approximately 45 minutes from my previous time despite still employing a combination of running and walking. Although I again had cramping, the experience allowed me further refine my understanding of my body's capabilities.

Continuing with my nutrition regimen, I gradually gained an understanding of what my body could and could not tolerate. In the same year, I participated in the Woodlands half marathon in March and the Houston half marathon in October, mirroring my activities from the previous year. Through these experiences, I began to discern patterns in how my body responded to different activities and dietary choices.

By 2021, I had a better and deeper understanding of my body's needs. I realized that activities lasting less than two hours better suited my fitness level and nutritional intake. Drawing from research related to nutrition and energy use, I learned more about energy metabolism, particularly focusing on how the body converts fats into energy and the role of stored glycogen in the liver.

During prolonged exercise, such as marathon running, the body relies heavily on stored fats for fuel, especially as glycogen stores become depleted. This process, known as fatty acid oxidation, allows the body to sustain endurance over extended durations.

However, I also learned that the availability of glucose, derived from carbohydrates, plays a crucial role in supporting high-intensity activities and maintaining optimal performance. As glycogen stores diminish during prolonged exercise, maintaining a steady supply of glucose becomes essential for sustaining energy levels and preventing fatigue. With this knowledge, I strategically tailored my nutrition and training approach to match my body's responses and optimize performance and energy utilization.

Scientific research supports the notion that during high-intensity activities lasting less than two hours, the body predominantly utilizes carbohydrates, stored as glycogen in muscles and the liver, as its primary energy source. According to the American College of Sports Medicine, fat becomes a more significant energy source during prolonged, lower-intensity exercise (ACSM, 2016). This insight led me to concentrate on shorter endurance events, like half marathons, which align with this metabolic characteristic, allowing for an optimal balance between endurance and energy expenditure. This strategic shift suited my body's natural energy utilization patterns and enabled me to tailor my training and nutritional plans more effectively for these specific types of events.

By concentrating on activities within this timeframe, I could capitalize on my body's ability to efficiently utilize fat stores while ensuring an adequate supply of glucose to support sustained effort. This approach helped me maintain energy levels throughout the race and facilitated quicker recovery post-event.

As a result, I've prioritized participation in half marathon races, as they align with my understanding of energy metabolism and performance optimization. This strategic approach has allowed me to sustain my fitness levels and achieve consistent results in my athletic efforts since 2021. In fact, I've already completed four half marathons in 2024, one each in January, February, March, and April.

Thus, for me, setting my personal health and fitness goals during the transition to the OMAD lifestyle involved a deliberate process of identifying ambitious objectives and understanding the right nutrition intake.

SETTING SMART GOALS

It's essential to ensure that your objectives are SMART—specific, measurable, achievable, relevant, and time-bound. By adhering to this framework, you can effectively align your aspirations with the principles of the OMAD lifestyle.

Firstly, it's crucial to establish specific goals that provide clarity and focus. This involves defining precise outcomes that reflect desired achievements within the context of the OMAD regimen. For example, rather than simply aiming to "improve fitness," a specific goal could be to "complete a half marathon within a specified timeframe."

Next, incorporating measurable elements will allow you to track progress and evaluate your success objectively. This entails quantifying goals in terms of distance, time, or other relevant metrics. For instance, setting a target time to complete a half marathon provides a clear benchmark for progress assessment.

Moreover, goals should be achievable, considering personal capabilities and constraints. Setting realistic objectives helps maintain motivation and sustain efforts over time. Considering your current fitness levels and available resources can help you tailor your goals to your circumstances.

Relevance is key to ensuring that goals are meaningful and aligned with personal values and priorities. Goals should resonate with you and contribute to your overall well-being and fulfillment. For example, pursuing fitness goals that enhance physical health and vitality aligns with optimizing health through the OMAD lifestyle.

Finally, incorporating a time-bound element adds a sense of urgency and accountability to goals, facilitating progress and preventing delay. Establishing clear deadlines or milestones can help you stay on track and maintain momentum toward your objectives. For example, setting a target date for completing a half marathon provides a timeframe for training and preparation.

My SMART Framework to Achieve Professional and Physical Wellness Goals

I approached my goals from multiple dimensions to ensure they were SMART—specific, measurable, achievable, relevant, and time-bound.

Firstly, regarding my professional sphere within the energy industry, I dedicated myself to optimizing work hours and focusing on performance metrics. The sector is cyclical, often experiencing phases where the demand for energy declines, leading to reduced workloads and, unfortunately, layoffs. Yet, I retained confidence in my skillset and capability to deliver high-quality work. I was determined to perform at a level that met my own high standards, ensuring that my contributions remained valuable and impactful, regardless of the industry's fluctuations.

From a physical and exercise perspective, I set measurable objectives related to running races and completing them satisfactorily. Reflecting on past challenges and struggles, I identified areas for improvement and sought to overcome them through targeted preparation and training. By specifying the criteria for success and observing tangible progress over time, I ensured that my goals were both measurable and achievable.

Moreover, the relevance of my goals was evident in their alignment with my overarching aspirations for health and fitness. Recognizing the transformative impact of my lifestyle changes, I prioritized goals that contributed to my overall well-being and personal growth. This ensured that my efforts remained focused on meaningful and impactful objectives in the context of my journey.

Lastly, I established time-bound goals that provided a clear framework for action and evaluation. By setting deadlines and milestones for both professional and fitness-related objectives, I created a sense of urgency and accountability. This enabled me to track progress effectively and adjust my approach to stay on course toward achieving my goals.

Thus, by following the SMART criteria, I created goals tailored to the one-meal-a-day lifestyle, promoting success and sustainability in my health and fitness attempts.

Measuring Incremental Progress and Celebrating Milestones

Measuring progress along my journey involved a combination of methods, each providing valuable insights into my performance and development. One key approach was maintaining written records, which allowed me to track my achievements and assess my progress over time. By documenting my experiences in both work and exercise, I gained clarity on areas where I excelled and areas where I could improve.

By returning to basics and using pen and paper, I could document my progress, accomplishments, and actions in my own handwriting. This record served as a visual reminder of what I had achieved and how I had approached my meals and activities.

Writing out details, such as the specific meals consumed and the corresponding physical activities undertaken, allowed me to gain clarity and insight into my lifestyle choices. These details on paper provided a clear picture of my daily habits and behaviors.

Moreover, the act of documenting my journey was like a form of self-accountability. When reviewing my entries, I naturally felt compelled to reflect on my experiences and consider areas for improvement. This process of self-reflection and goal-setting encouraged a continuous cycle of growth and progress.

Additionally, monitoring my energy levels served as a reliable indicator of my overall well-being and fitness. Observing fluctuations in energy throughout the day provided valuable feedback on the effectiveness of my lifestyle choices and helped me adjust accordingly.

Celebrating milestones was an essential aspect of staying motivated and recognizing my accomplishments. Receiving medals for completing races served as reminders of my progress and provided a sense of achievement. Each medal represented a milestone in my journey, signifying the dedication and effort I invested to achieve my goals.

Furthermore, I used various exercise apps and tools to track my performance during workouts. These resources offered valuable metrics such as pace, heart rate, and VO2 max, allowing me to measure my progress and identify areas for improvement. I could see evidence of my growth and development by comparing my performance over time.

The combination of written records, energy monitoring, race medals, and exercise metrics provided a comprehensive framework for measuring incremental progress and celebrating milestones along my journey toward health and fitness.

Celebrating milestones along my journey is a powerful source of motivation and reinforcement of my long-term objectives. Initially, these celebrations were personal, where I reflected on the moments and engaged in self-recognition for the progress I achieved. However, as I integrated others into my fitness goals, we started celebrating together, bringing friends and family along for the journey.

Sharing my achievements with others allowed me to inspire and motivate them to pursue their own health and fitness goals. As friends and family joined me in activities like running half marathons, we bonded over shared experiences and accomplishments. Together, we celebrated each milestone reached, fostering a sense of connection and support that fueled our collective progress.

While many people readily embraced the exercise aspect of my journey, I recognized the opportunity to raise awareness about the crucial role of nutrition in achieving overall well-being. By showcasing the integration of nutrition and fitness, I aim to provide a holistic understanding of health and inspire others to prioritize both aspects of their lives.

3

BALANCED NUTRIENT-DENSE DIET

The one-meal-a-day lifestyle is a commitment to transforming how we think about food, its timing, and its impact on our overall health. Through this chapter, I will guide you through the critical aspects of nutrition and meal planning, emphasizing the need for careful consideration and understanding of our eating habits. It aims to shed light on creating balanced, nutritious meals that cater to our physical needs and our mental and emotional well-being.

Transitioning to the OMAD lifestyle requires more than just the willpower to eat once a day; it demands a strategic approach to selecting what we eat. The journey to success involves balancing macronutrients, ensuring adequate micronutrient intake, and recognizing how food influences our mood and cognitive functions.

In this detailed exploration, I'll dive into the principles of nutritional planning tailored to the OMAD framework, sharing insights from personal experiences, practical tips, and my favorites. Understanding these foundational elements will enhance your appreciation of the connection between diet and quality of life, ensuring that your OMAD journey is nutritionally rewarding as well as life-enhancing.

MOTIVATION AND MOOD AWARENESS

Embracing the one-meal-a-day (OMAD) lifestyle was not a deliberate choice initially but was primarily motivated by the noticeable boost in the mental clarity, attention, and focus I experienced from adjusting my meal times. This significant improvement in cognitive function underpinned my decision to continue with the change in eating and finally adopt OMAD, focusing on what I eat and when. However, it took a few years.

In the early stages of this dietary shift, my choices regarding the day's first meal were less about nutritional quality and more about convenience. It was a practical decision, driven by the immediate need to eat after extended periods of fasting. However, as I progressed, I started noticing a pattern in the direct link between the foods I consumed and my mood fluctuations. This observation led to a deeper understanding of 'mood awareness'—recognizing the impact of dietary choices on my emotional well-being.

However, this awareness didn't develop overnight. Over the years, as I gradually shifted towards prioritizing quality foods, I started incorporating salads and proteins into my first meal. This change maintained and enhanced my mental clarity, changing my dietary approach. Unlike before, when my focus might have waned with other food choices, nutrient-rich meals such as salads fortified with proteins supported my cognitive functions more effectively.

This transition to selecting quality, nutritious foods was gradual but deliberate, reflecting a broader understanding of how diet influences physical health and mental and emotional states. I discovered that the path to sustaining mental clarity and focus through OMAD lies in the careful consideration of not just the timing but food quality.

NUTRITIONAL GUIDELINES

Adopting the OMAD approach required a deliberate shift in how I approached my diet, where I had to do considerable dietary refinement. Through a structured progression of stages, I focused on elevating the nutritional value of my meals. Initially, this process involved integrating more wholesome, nutritious foods into my daily eating plan, setting a foundation for the comprehensive nutritional strategy that unfolded later. This methodical progression allowed me to gradually enhance the quality of my meals, laying the groundwork for a sophisticated and holistic approach to nutrition.

Phase 1: Embracing Convenience with a Nutritional Mindset

In the initial six months of my transition to healthier eating, I focused on integrating more vegetables and lean proteins into my diet that suited my busy lifestyle. This phase saw me opt for ready-to-eat options available at the grocery store, such as pre-packed vegetables and rotisserie chicken. These convenient choices, including coleslaw and mixed salads with dressing, were my go-to foods for breaking the fast. They provided a straightforward way to consume vegetables without the need for preparation.

However, my commitment to better nutrition went beyond the convenient options. I made sure to include a variety of vegetables, like red cabbage, white cabbage, and carrots, alongside cucumbers and cilantro, ensuring a diverse intake of nutrients. Avocados became a staple for their healthy fats. I complemented these vegetable-based meals with fruits such as bananas, aiming for a balanced mix of vitamins, minerals, and other essential nutrients.

This approach marked my first steps towards a more health-conscious lifestyle. By choosing foods that were both convenient and nutritious, I stepped forward toward more complex meal planning and preparation. Including a broad range of vegetables, the healthy fats from avocados, and the natural sugars and additional vitamins from fruits like bananas set the stage for the next phases of my nutritional journey. This phase was instrumental in teaching me the importance of making thoughtful food choices, even within the constraints of a busy schedule, paving the way for more elaborate meal planning as my journey progressed.

Phase 2: Home-Cooked Meals

Moving into the second phase of my nutritional planning, I embraced the hands-on approach of preparing my own meals. This step marked a significant shift towards a more intentional and health-focused dietary regimen. I expanded my use of fresh vegetables, which I had initially started eating. Avocados continued to be a crucial part of my diet for their healthy fats and nutrient density, along with oven-baked slices of potatoes, enriching my meals with their complex carbohydrates.

During this phase, grilling became a preferred method to cook lean proteins without compromising taste or nutritional value. I grilled chicken and fish, chosen for their lean quality and the essential proteins they provided. The grilling technique effectively preserves the nutritional value of these proteins while ensuring the meals remain flavorful.

I also started broadening my carbohydrate sources by including boiled potatoes, sweet potatoes, and plantains, each offering a rich source of energy and dietary fiber. Introducing plantains to my diet brought diversity to my carbohydrate intake and added a unique flavor to my meals. Alongside these, I prepared separate vegetable dishes featuring broccoli and cauliflower, ensuring each meal was balanced with greens loaded with vitamins, minerals, and antioxidants. The protein portion of my meals also expanded to a variety of seafood.

This phase was marked by a deliberate balance of macronutrients and an enhanced focus on micronutrient-rich vegetables and fruits, laying the groundwork for a nutritionally robust OMAD diet.

Phase 3: Enhancing Diet with Complex Carbs and Seafood

Progressing into the next phase of my dietary planning, I focused on enriching my meals with a wider array of complex carbohydrates and diversifying my protein sources, particularly through an increased seafood intake. This period was characterized by a more fine approach to balancing my diet, ensuring it was both nutrient-dense and fulfilling.

I incorporated boiled potatoes, including both sweet potatoes and smaller ones known as "baby potatoes," alongside plantains, into my meals. These sources of complex carbohydrates provided sustained energy and were vital for maintaining my physical health. Additionally, I started preparing separate vegetable dishes featuring broccoli and cauliflower, aiming to enhance my meals with fiber, vitamins, and minerals essential for optimal health.

The introduction of a variety of seafood—including fish, shrimp, and occasionally scallops—allowed me to benefit from high-quality proteins and the omega-3 fatty acids they offer. This shift diversified my nutrient intake and added new flavors and textures to my meals, making them more satisfying.

Avocados remained a constant in my diet for their healthy fats. Not to mention, water continued to be my primary drink, ensuring I stayed well-hydrated. Fruits and vegetables rounded out my meals, providing a spectrum of micronutrients and antioxidants to support overall wellness.

This phase marked a deliberate effort to craft a balanced and healthful eating plan within the OMAD framework. By focusing on the quality of carbohydrates, incorporating various protein sources, and maintaining a rich intake of fruits and vegetables, I created meals that supported my health goals and accommodated my evolving dietary preferences.

Phase 4: Experimenting with Vegetarian Options

In the fourth phase of my nutritional journey, I transitioned to a vegetarian diet. I shifted towards using legumes as my primary protein source. Lentils, black-eyed peas, and chickpeas became central to my diet, serving as versatile and nutritious alternatives to animal proteins. This transition was enhanced by combining these legumes with a colorful array of bell peppers—red, orange, yellow, and green—along with onions and tomatoes. This mix, seasoned with well-chosen spices, created flavorful and protein-rich dishes that were both satisfying and aligned with vegetarian principles.

In this phase, I continued to include plantains and a variety of potatoes as my main sources of carbohydrates, maintaining the energy levels required for my daily activities. The vegetables that had become staples in my diet, such as broccoli, cauliflower, and carrots, remained essential, ensuring my meals were balanced and rich.

Water remained my hydration of choice, vital for supporting the body's processes, including digestion and nutrient absorption. Fruits also played a significant role, providing natural sugars, additional fiber, and a range of micronutrients that complemented vegetarian meals.

This exploration into vegetarianism wasn't just a dietary adjustment but a period of significant learning and experimentation. It allowed me to delve deeper into the nutritional possibilities of plant-based eating, understanding the importance of combining different foods to fully meet my nutritional needs. While this phase wasn't permanent, it broadened my perspective on diet and health, enriching my knowledge of how diverse vegetarian meals could support my lifestyle and well-being.

Phase 5: Embracing a Mixed Diet Approach

In the fifth and last phase of dietary evolution, I transitioned back to a mixed diet approach. This comprehensive strategy incorporated a broad spectrum of foods: a variety of meats, emphasizing lean options like chicken and a range of seafood while consciously avoiding high-fat proteins such as pork. This approach was a significant deviation from my initial reliance on pre-packed foods, signaling a more mature phase of dietary planning.

For groceries, the list was simple, divided into categories to ensure all aspects of my nutritional needs were covered. Proteins included options like shrimp, salmon, and chicken, reflecting my preference for leaner meats and seafood. For carbohydrates, I opted for plantains and both sweet and regular potatoes.

Avocados became my go-to source of healthy fats, versatile enough to complement any meal. I supplemented them with olive oil for cooking and dressing. My fruit and vegetable selection remained versatile, mainly including apples, bananas, peaches, cauliflower, broccoli, and carrots.

The 'others' category in my list included essentials like coffee and water, with the addition of treats such as dark chocolate and a mix of nuts, including peanuts, cashews, and Brazil nuts, adding taste and nutritional variety to my diet.

This structured approach to meal planning allowed me to maintain a balanced diet that was both satisfying and aligned with my health goals. By carefully selecting a range of foods from each category, I ensured my OMAD diet was nutrient-dense and macro and micronutrient-balanced, supporting my physical and mental health. This phase was about applying the lessons learned throughout my journey to achieve a harmonious and flexible eating plan that catered to my evolving dietary preferences and lifestyle.

Spices-Tailoring Flavors to Nutrition

In adjusting my one-meal-a-day diet, I've come to value the role of spices for taste. While planning your meal, remember that food should be both enjoyable and nutritious. Spices allow you to personalize your meals and keep your diet interesting and aligned with your health goals.

My selection is brief, focusing on around six spices that I find essential for enhancing flavor. My go-to choices are seasoned salt, powdered onions, oregano, basil, black pepper, and salt. These staples bring out the best in any dish, enhancing flavors without overshadowing the natural taste of fresh ingredients. While this is my foundational spice palette, you can explore and expand your spice list based on personal preference and nutritional goals.

For those looking to diversify their seasoning repertoire, consider incorporating spices like turmeric, cinnamon, and cumin. Garlic powder, though not on my essential list, can add a robust flavor and boost immunity. Each spice contributes a unique flavor profile and offers distinct health benefits, making your meal a culinary delight and a nutritional powerhouse.

STREAMLINING MEAL PREPARATION: EFFICIENCY, NUTRITION, AND ADAPTABILITY

My grocery shopping became strategic and intentional, organized around creating a balanced and diverse one-meal-a-day diet. Organizing my list into specific categories streamlined my shopping process significantly, allowing me to finish and come out of the grocery store efficiently, often within 15 minutes. This efficiency was built on an earlier routine where I focused on selecting pre-packed vegetables and rotisserie chicken, which provided a straightforward, nutritious option for breaking my fast. These choices ensured I had immediate access to high-energy and healthy foods, including avocados and several fruits and vegetables.

I not only saved time but also transitioned into more deliberate meal planning. As my dietary focus shifted, I found it straightforward to select the right types of vegetables and lean meat for grilling, which aligned with my evolving nutritional goals. My grocery list, carefully divided into proteins, carbohydrates, fats, fruits, vegetables, and other essentials, became a tool for maintaining a balanced diet from Monday to Friday. This system supported a lifestyle that prioritized my health without compromising convenience.

As I became more adept at navigating my meal-a-day lifestyle, I discovered that preparing a nutritious, high-quality meal was surprisingly efficient, often taking less than 30 minutes. This revelation came from streamlining my meal prep process, which involves some initial preparation but significantly reduces cooking time. This efficiency ensures that, even on the busiest of days, a wholesome meal is within reach shortly after I return home.

For those moments when hunger is more pressing, I found that snacking on fruits is a quick and healthy solution to tide me over the cooking period. This practice underlines the importance of readily available nutritious snacks, aligning with the overall goal of maintaining a balanced diet.

I advocate for developing a meal preparation system that suits your lifestyle and dietary preferences. Initially, it's beneficial to personally select and prepare your foods, familiarize yourself with the process, and understand the nutritional value of different ingredients. Over time, this knowledge allows for flexibility, such as delegating meal preparation, making informed choices when dining out, or attending social events.

This approach to meal planning is about nurturing a healthy relationship with food, understanding its preparation, and enjoying the variety it brings to your life. Whether you're cooking for yourself or choosing meals in other settings, the key is consistently making choices that support your health goals. This overview encapsulates the essence of meal planning within the OMAD framework, emphasizing simplicity, nutrition, and adaptability.

SAMPLE MENUS AND RECIPES

Diverse Meal Ideas

Ensuring a varied diet within the one-meal-a-day (OMAD) lifestyle involves strategic planning and creativity in meal preparation. When it comes to meal preparation, it's crucial to communicate the variety and foundation of the dietary approach I advocate. I have built this foundation on a set of go-to meals designed for ease and convenience, offering a simple alternative to the typical choices of the standard American diet—be it grabbing a hamburger, pizza, or tacos.

To accommodate different tastes while staying true to a meal-a-day approach, I've developed a method of diversifying my meals by applying different cooking techniques and combinations to a set of core ingredients. This strategy keeps the meals interesting and palatable and ensures nutritional adequacy. At the most basic level, I have identified seven core meals, each constructed around simplicity and nutritional balance, akin to having a well-rounded plate that could include chicken, seafood, potatoes, broccoli, and avocados.

Using a basic assortment of 10 ingredients, it's possible to create an array of meals that span the entire week, demonstrating the flexibility of the OMAD lifestyle. For illustration, here's a list of ingredients I use to create five distinct meals:

Core Ingredients

- Salmon (2 pieces)
- Chicken breast (3 pieces)
- Avocados
- Sweet potatoes
- Russet potatoes
- Broccoli
- Cucumber
- Cauliflower
- Carrots
- Seasoning

Meal Plans

Meal 1:
- **Chicken:** Grilled with seasoning for a flavorful main.
- **Sweet Potatoes:** Boiled, seasoned, then lightly fried for a balanced taste.
- **Cauliflower and Broccoli:** Stir-fried with seasoning for added texture.
- **Avocados:** Included fresh to complement the dish with healthy fats.

Meal 2:

- **Chicken:** Diced, seasoned, boiled, and then given a light fry for tenderness.
- **Sweet Potatoes:** Thinly sliced, seasoned, and oven-baked for crispness.
- **Cauliflower and Broccoli:** Oven-baked with seasoning for a different flavor profile.
- **Avocados:** Provided to enrich the meal with nutrients and smoothness.

Meal 3:
- **Salmon:** Seasoned, cut, boiled, and lightly fried for a delicate flavor.
- **Russet Potatoes:** Boiled and seasoned to serve as a hearty side.
- **Cauliflower and Broccoli:** Finely chopped, seasoned, and fried for variety in texture.
- **Avocados:** Added for their creamy texture and health benefits.

Meal 4:
- **Salmon:** Seasoned and oven-baked, providing a rich taste.
- **Sweet Potatoes:** Boiled, seasoned, and then lightly fried for flavor.
- **Cauliflower and Broccoli:** Stir-fried with seasoning to enhance the meal.
- **Avocados:** Freshly included, offering a smooth and healthy addition to the dish.

Meal 5:
- **Mixed Vegetables:** Cucumber, carrots, broccoli, and more, chopped and dressed with avocado for a refreshing salad.
- **Salmon and Chicken:** Both boiled and oven-baked, offering a hearty and nutritious protein selection.

Through such variations, this lifestyle can support a wide range of dietary preferences, including vegetarian options, by utilizing the same foundational ingredients in several innovative ways.

The idea is to consider a typical meal that embodies the principles of the OMAD lifestyle while catering to an active lifestyle. Such a meal would feature two chicken breasts as the protein anchor, complemented by two sizable russet potatoes and one or two heads of broccoli. This combination delivers essential proteins and a rich array of nutrients and fiber, with the addition of two avocados introducing beneficial fats and a creamy texture that enhances the overall meal.

The success of this meal hinges on a well-thought-out grocery list and a straightforward recipe. For someone following my approach, the shopping list will include the specific quantities mentioned: approximately two pounds of chicken (or about two chicken breasts), ensuring the protein portion of the meal is ample, and the inclusion of two large russet potatoes, two avocados, and a couple of heads of broccoli. You may have noticed that I use everything in two. It is because I've found that this methodical approach to portioning ensures each meal is both satisfying and aligned with nutritional goals.

In terms of hydration, incorporating two 16-ounce water bottles ensures adequate fluid intake, summing up to 32 ounces. A cup of olive oil is suggested for cooking, providing a healthy fat source that enhances the meal's flavor and nutritional profile. The seasoning mix, key for elevating the taste, could consist of two tablespoons each of salt and black pepper, alongside a tablespoon each of ground onion, rosemary, oregano, and an optional tablespoon of basil or any preferred herb, illustrating the customization available in tailoring each meal to individual taste preferences.

This detailed approach to organizing meals under the OMAD lifestyle highlights the importance of selecting quality ingredients and preparing them in a convenient and nourishing manner. It promotes a conscious relationship with food, focusing on each component's integrity and nutritional content.

Advanced Meal Preparation Techniques

While discussing the diverse meal ideas within the OMAD framework, it's essential to delve deeper into the meal preparation methods that emphasize convenience, nutritional balance, and taste variety. My own approach to selecting, seasoning, and mixing different ingredients has been instrumental in enriching my OMAD journey. This personalized exploration into meal prep has been key to aligning my daily intake with my health and wellness objectives, showcasing this lifestyle's capacity for flexibility and personal adaptation.

Foundational Meal Preparation

A fundamental meal setup may include a balanced combination of proteins, carbohydrates, vegetables, and healthy fats. For instance, a meal incorporating chicken, russet potatoes, broccoli, and avocados has a comprehensive nutrient profile. The preparation process involves separately cooking each component to retain its distinct flavors and nutritional benefits:

- **Chicken and Vegetables:** The chicken is sliced or diced and cooked in a pot with water and a blend of seasonings, including salt, pepper, ground onion, rosemary, oregano, and optionally basil. Feel free to add more spices based on your taste preferences, allowing for a personalized flavor profile that caters to your individual palate. Apply the same seasoning to the vegetables, ensuring a harmonious flavor throughout the dish. After boiling, the chicken is stir-fried in olive oil to

achieve the desired taste, and the vegetables are mixed in to create a flavorful stir-fry.
- **Potatoes:** Russet potatoes are sliced and boiled in a separate pot, then optionally tossed with a bit of olive oil and parsley for added flavor.

This base method of meal preparation is adaptable and can be elaborated upon depending on an individual'spersonal preferences or dietary needs.

Alternative Ingredients for Variety

- The protein source can be diverse by substituting chicken with shrimp or other seafood, adjusting the quantity to match dietary requirements.
- Similarly, russet potatoes can be replaced with sweet potatoes and broccoli with other vegetables like cauliflower, eggplant, or cabbage, following the same foundational cooking and seasoning principles.

Cooking Methods and Timing

These meals can be prepared using various cooking methods—on the burner, grilled, or baked—with the cooking time adjusted accordingly. For burner cooking, meals can be prepared in as little as 15 minutes, while oven and grill methods may extend the cooking time but often enhance flavor.

Introducing Fruits and Vegetarian Options

- The integration of fruits, such as sliced apples, grapes, or pears, at the beginning of the meal can provide a refreshing start, especially when breaking the OMAD fast.
- For a vegetarian alternative, lentils are an excellent protein base, cooked with a stew made from tomatoes, bell peppers, onions, and a similar seasoning blend. This

combination is cooked until the lentils are tender, with vegetables and carbohydrates like potatoes or sweet potatoes rounding off the meal.

Meal Customization

The art of meal preparation within OMAD lies in adjusting the seasoning and components to suit individual taste preferences, ensuring the meal is as enjoyable as it is nutritious. This flexibility allows for a personalized eating experience, catering to individuals' diverse tastes and nutritional needs following the OMAD lifestyle.

These advanced meal preparation techniques highlight the importance of a structured yet flexible approach to cooking within the OMAD diet and how a thoughtful selection of ingredients and cooking methods can lead to meals that are both enjoyable and supportive of an active lifestyle, including participation in activities as demanding as a half marathon.

Nutritional Planning and Adaptation Strategies

Integrating Dietary Restrictions and Preferences

When tailoring common meals to fit the OMAD lifestyle, especially for individuals with specific dietary restrictions or preferences, the primary goal is to create a balanced, nutrient-dense diet. The key strategy involves breaking down a meal into its constituent ingredients across the major nutritional categories: proteins, carbohydrates, fats, fruits, vegetables, and others. For example, a hamburger typically comprises protein (the meat), carbohydrates (the bun), and vegetables (lettuce). The goal here is to consider how one can modify this common meal to enhance its nutritional density, choosing better options that still align with one's personal dietary restrictions and preferences.

This approach emphasizes the importance of being mindful of meal composition, encouraging individuals to make informed decisions that cater to their dietary needs and contribute to a nutrient-dense diet. The objective is to ensure that every meal, even within the OMAD framework, is as nutritious as possible, supporting an active and healthy lifestyle.

By raising awareness of how small adjustments to meal components can create more nutritionally complete choices, I aim to empower everyone to make dietary changes that enhance their overall health. This guidance is particularly relevant for adapting common meals to fit the OMAD lifestyle, ensuring that each meal provides a balanced array of nutrients essential for sustaining energy levels and promoting well-being.

Strategic Ingredient Replacement

Upon identifying nutritional gaps, strategic replacements are necessary to ensure the meal remains aligned with the OMAD framework while catering to dietary needs:

- **Complex for Simple:** Substitute simple carbohydrates with complex alternatives to enhance the meal's nutritional profile and provide sustained energy release.
- **Lean for Fatty:** Opt for lean protein sources over fatty ones, improving the meal's overall health without compromising protein quality.

This approach facilitates a comprehensive nutritional intake and effectively accommodates specific dietary requirements. By visually laying out the meal's components, individuals can easily adjust their meal plans to avoid nutrient deficiencies, ensuring their one daily meal is both satisfying and conducive to an active lifestyle.

Supporting an Active Lifestyle

It's crucial to remember that the OMAD lifestyle aims to provide sufficient energy and nutrients to support rigorous exercise and maintain vitality. Therefore, every meal should be constructed with this goal in mind, using the strategy of ingredient categorization and replacement to tailor meals that meet these rigorous demands.

FAVORITE MEALS AND ADAPTING FOUNDATION RECIPES

Crafting Foundation Meals within the OMAD Framework

In my journey through the OMAD lifestyle, I've developed a repertoire of meals that form the cornerstone of my dietary approach. This foundational structure, critical to maintaining nutritional balance and variety, supports an active lifestyle while adhering to the OMAD principles. Below is a glimpse into this foundation, showcasing the diversity and adaptability of the meals I've integrated into my routine.

Foundation Meals Overview

- **Beef-Based Meal** features tender beef chunks paired with an assortment of vegetables, complemented by potatoes for a hearty source of carbohydrates and avocados for healthy fats.

- **Chicken-Centric Meal** consists of well-seasoned chicken, served alongside a variety of vegetables, potatoes for sustenance, and avocados to enrich the meal with their creamy texture and nutritional benefits.

- **Salmon Centerpiece Meal** highlights salmon as the protein focus, accompanied by vegetables and plantain for a balance of flavors, with avocados adding a smooth finish to the dish.

- **Lentil-Based Meal** showcases lentils paired with a rich stew, vegetables for added micronutrients, sweet potatoes as a complex carbohydrate source, and avocados for their versatility and healthful fats.

- **Quinoa as a Core Ingredient** features quinoa accompanied by a flavorful stew, a mix of vegetables, sweet potatoes for energy, and avocados to round off the meal with its nutritional profile.
- **Egg-Centric Meal** includes eggs as a protein staple, combined with vegetables and sweet potatoes for a well-rounded dish, enhanced by the inclusion of plantains and an avocado dressing for extra flavor and nutrition.

Integrating Personal Favorites and Meal Adaptation

Building on this foundation, I've found meals that meet the OMAD criteria nourishing and scrumptious, and they've become my personal favorites due to their flavor, nutritional content, and satisfaction. Among these, a versatile and nutrient-packed salad stands out as a refreshing yet fulfilling option that has sustained me for extended periods.

The Composition of a Staple Salad

- **Base:** The salad includes a generous mix of red and white cabbage, chopped into bite-sized pieces, forming the leafy, colorful foundation of the meal.
- **Additions:** To this, I add a large, peeled, and chopped cucumber for freshness alongside chopped carrots for a slight sweetness and crunch. A sprinkle of corn and a garnish of cilantro add layers of texture and flavor.
- **Dressing:** The salad is brought together with a homemade dressing—a blend of avocados, olive oil, habanero pepper for a bit of heat, salt, and pepper, all mixed into a creamy paste that envelopes each ingredient in rich flavor.

Protein Options

- **Fish:** Grilled or boiled, then stir-fried fish, seasoned with a basic yet effective blend of spices, serves as a lean protein source complementing the salad.
- **Eggs:** Alternatively, four to six boiled eggs, peeled, can be included for protein, offering a different texture and taste to the meal.

Satisfying Sides

- **Carbohydrates:** For an additional carbohydrate source, thinly sliced plantains or potatoes, seasoned with salt, pepper, and a touch of olive oil, then oven-baked until crisp, making a delightful side that rounds off the meal.

Customization and Variety

This salad and its accompaniments highlight the principle of customization within the OMAD lifestyle. Just as some might enjoy a hamburger for several consecutive days, the body can also grow to crave and relish this nutrient-dense salad. However, the beauty of such a foundational meal lies in its potential for variation. The same ingredients can be slightly altered or cooked differently—such as stir-frying the salad mix with various seasonings—to introduce a new flavor profile and prevent monotony.

Foundation for Creativity

These foundational meals are staples in my diet and serve as a basis for creativity and experimentation in the kitchen. By starting with a solid nutritional base and allowing for modifications, I can ensure my meals remain exciting and diverse. This approach emphasizes the importance of a versatile and enriching foundation that supports an active lifestyle and caters to the body's needs during the OMAD journey.

OPTIMIZING PRE-RACE NUTRITION WITHIN THE OMAD FRAMEWORK

Tailoring Meals for Athletic Performance

In health and fitness, especially when gearing up for athletic competitions like races, the composition of the pre-event meal becomes crucial. My approach to this vital meal has evolved, embodying the principles of the OMAD lifestyle while specifically targeting performance and endurance enhancement.

A Pre-Race Meal Strategy

On the eve of race day, I focus on a meal designed to boost my energy levels and ensure optimal hydration. This meal includes:

- **Egg Whites Omelet:** A lean source of protein, prepared by removing the yolks and lightly frying the whites, similar to an omelet. This component is key for muscle repair and recovery.

- **Spinach:** Cooked separately, this leafy green is rich in iron and vitamins, facilitating oxygen transport throughout the body.

- **Chopped Vegetables:** Like my routine preparation of cauliflower and broccoli, these vegetables are chopped and cooked separately, providing essential nutrients to the body without heavy digestion.

- **Carbohydrates:** The intake of carbohydrates is liberal, focusing on eating until satisfaction to ensure stored energy is maximized for the upcoming physical exertion.

- **Hydration:** Drinking ample water the night before is necessary to maintain proper hydration levels.

This meal plan is about nourishing the body and mentally and physically preparing myself for the exertion to come. By morning, with only water and coffee to start the day, I find myself well-prepared and energized, ready to participate in the race or extended cycling sessions.

Application to Running and Cycling

This dietary strategy proves its versatility and effectiveness in endurance sports:

- **Running:** For activities like running, this meal plan supports sustained energy for up to two hours of continuous activity.
- **Cycling:** For cycling, especially at lower intensities, the same OMAD principles allow for up to five hours of activity without the need for in-exercise nutrition, focusing on post-exercise replenishment instead.

This pre-race nutrition approach within the OMAD lifestyle highlights the possibility of achieving significant health and fitness milestones. By thoughtfully selecting and timing meals to precede athletic endeavors, it's possible to enhance performance, endurance, and overall physical readiness, all while adhering to the OMAD principles. This strategy caters to the immediate needs of the race day and aligns with long-term health and wellness goals as well, illustrating the adaptability of the OMAD diet to support active lifestyles across various sports disciplines.

For an in-depth exploration of how the OMAD lifestyle has supported my athletic achievements across numerous running and cycling events over five years, please refer to Chapter 7, '*Documenting the Journey*'. This chapter provides a comprehensive look at the milestones I reached exclusively through adherence to the OMAD principles, showcasing the diet's impact on my sustained athletic performance and lifestyle transformation.

Meal Success through Nutritional Density and Exercise Support

Reflecting on the meals that stand out as significant successes in terms of nutritional content and overall satisfaction, I invariably return to the foundation meals I've curated. These meals are distinguished by their nutritional density and adeptness in supporting vigorous exercise routines. Each foundation meal reflects nutritional completeness and is carefully composed to include a broad range of micro and macronutrients. This comprehensiveness turns each meal into a powerhouse of energy and sustenance, precisely meeting my dietary requirements and enhancing overall health.

The efficacy of these meals also stems from their ability to achieve a balanced mix of essential nutrients. Providing an optimal blend of proteins, carbohydrates, fats, vitamins, and minerals ensures the body is fueled sufficiently for everyday activities as well as for more demanding physical challenges.

Perhaps the most significant measure of these meals' success is their role in facilitating rigorous exercise regimes. The nutritional groundwork laid by these meals is specially tailored for athletic performance, allowing for prolonged physical activity without taxing the body excessively. This capability to support extensive workouts without leading to nutritional deficits or physical exhaustion emphasizes the effectiveness of the foundational meals in promoting an active, healthy lifestyle.

CRAFTING A WEEKLY MEAL PLAN

Approaching meal planning for the week, especially within the OMAD lifestyle's constraints, centers significantly around thoughtful preparation and adaptability. The cornerstone of this process is developing a detailed grocery list, tailored to the specific meals envisioned for the week. The aim is to strike a balance, maintaining consistency in nutritional intake from

Monday to Friday while also embracing flexibility during weekends and holidays. This approach emphasizes that adapting to the OMAD lifestyle isn't a rigid, all-or-nothing proposition but a gradual journey toward nutritional optimization and lifestyle adjustment.

Flexibility and Consistency Within the OMAD Lifestyle

I want to convey to my readers that adopting this lifestyle isn't a matter of black or white. Keep in mind, it requires time for your body to adjust, and this principle holds true for everyone, particularly my target audience.

Each person leads a distinct lifestyle, and acknowledging the diversity in their daily routines and activity levels is crucial. While some may lead exceptionally active lives, others might have more sedentary professional commitments. Yet, the commonality lies in their capacity for reasoned thought and an understanding of the scientific principles underpinning the OMAD approach.

This lifestyle is accessible to everyone, including those new to it, by employing a step-by-step method to condense their eating window slowly without drastic meal skipping. Instead of eliminating breakfast or dinner outright, the strategy involves delaying meals incrementally to observe the benefits, thereby naturally reducing unnecessary snacking and unhealthy habits.

From Gradual Shifts to Nutritional Density

Beginners, starting with small adjustments such as postponing a meal by 30 minutes, can see the advantages of this dietary shift, setting the stage for further modifications. This gradual narrowing of the eating window encourages a more mindful consumption of nutrient-dense foods, aligning dietary habits with personal health and fitness goals. Such a measured approach is especially beneficial for athletes, such as marathon runners, who might discover that the OMAD lifestyle enhances their metabolic efficiency, favoring fat utilization over glucose for energy.

Implementing Meal Planning

The practical steps to weekly meal planning within the OMAD framework involve:

1. Identifying the desired daily meals, focusing on nutritional balance and variety.
2. Writing down the components of these meals to visually map out the week's nutritional strategy.
3. Conducting focused grocery shopping based on this plan, ensuring all ingredients needed for the week's meals are procured.

This structured approach facilitates adherence to the OMAD lifestyle and ensures that each meal is a deliberate choice toward healthful living. It highlights the importance of planning and flexibility, allowing individuals to tailor their eating patterns to support an active lifestyle and achieve dietary satisfaction.

4

INTEGRATING EXERCISE

Exercise stands as a cornerstone of well-being, a truth universally acknowledged yet frequently overlooked in the pursuit of health. It is a critical component of a balanced lifestyle, offering extensive benefits that span the body's physical, mental, and emotional domains. As we delve deeper into the complex connection between physical activity and overall wellness, it becomes evident that exercise is not merely an adjunct to a healthy life but a fundamental element.

Following this foundational understanding of exercise's key role in health and well-being, this chapter aims to delve into the multifaceted benefits of exercise, particularly within the framework of the integrative OMAD lifestyle. Here, I aim to explore the advantages of exercise to physical and mental health as well as my personal journey of integrating exercise into my routine.

Through a detailed examination of scientific research and personal insights, this chapter will illuminate how the OMAD lifestyle enhances the efficacy of regular physical activity and vice versa, supporting metabolic health, improving mental clarity, and elevating the overall quality of life. By sharing this knowledge, I aspire to offer a comprehensive guide on incorporating exercise into your daily routine as an indispensable strategy for cultivating optimal health and well-being.

Let's study the multifaceted role of exercise, exploring the empirical evidence that supports its benefits and offering insights into effectively incorporating it into the fabric of our lives, all within the context of a balanced OMAD lifestyle.

BENEFITS OF EXERCISE IN THE LIGHT OF SCIENTIFIC EVIDENCE

Engaging in regular physical activity is essential for maintaining and improving health, offering numerous benefits across the physical, mental, and emotional health spectrums, the merits of which are well-documented and robust, underpinned by a wealth of scientific research.

Chronic Disease Prevention and Improved Cardiovascular Health

First, physical activity serves as a powerful barrier against many chronic diseases. Regular engagement in moderate to vigorous exercise is proven to significantly lower the risk of coronary heart disease, stroke, and type II diabetes. For example, running, as a form of physical activity, stands out for its extensive health benefits and accessibility. It's an efficient way to enhance cardiovascular health, improve body composition, and bolster mental well-being. Regular running sessions increase heart rate, promote blood circulation, and improve heart health.

Additionally, weight-bearing exercises, such as low-impact aerobics, walking, or running, help in managing cholesterol levels, further protecting against cardiovascular complications.

Moreover, it promises to extend life expectancy by reducing the risk of early death by as much as 30%.

Metabolic Health and Weight Management

From a metabolic perspective, it is an effective way to burn calories and fat, aiding in weight loss and management. It boosts the metabolic rate during the activity and for hours afterward, a phenomenon known as the afterburn effect or excess post-exercise oxygen consumption (EPOC). This makes running particularly beneficial for those seeking a leaner body composition.

Weight management is critical to maintaining overall health, with dietary habits and physical activity playing pivotal roles. The fundamental principle of weight management is the energy balance equation: to maintain a stable weight, the calories consumed through food and beverages must equal the calories expended through physical activity and metabolic processes. Conversely, for weight loss to occur, energy expenditure must exceed energy intake.

Achieving the recommended 150 minutes of moderate physical activity per week, which can include various activities such as running or walking, is essential for maintaining a healthy weight. It's important to note that individual needs for physical activity may vary significantly based on factors such as metabolic rate and body composition. For those looking to lose and sustain weight, an increased level of physical activity, coupled with adjustments to dietary intake to reduce calorie consumption, is necessary.

Research indicates that while exercise is crucial for weight management, it often requires more than the minimum recommended amounts to prevent weight gain or to achieve weight loss. This emphasizes the importance of engaging in regular physical activity and being mindful of dietary choices to avoid overestimating the calories burned through exercise.

Moreover, when I consider exercise, I remind myself of its role in weight management by burning calories and improving body composition, as evidenced by research. Recent research has shown that exercise reduces abdominal fat and supports weight control by enhancing lipid profiles—lowering serum triglyceride levels, increasing HDL (good) cholesterol, and reducing the LDL/HDL cholesterol ratio (Franczyk et al., 2023). Additionally, the evidence further indicates that it induces beneficial changes in lipoprotein subclasses, including a reduction in small, dense LDL particles and an increase in large LDL particles, which are associated with a reduced risk of cardiovascular diseases.

Mental Health Enhancement

Beyond its protective effects against physical ailments, the psychological benefits of exercise are equally compelling. It emerges as a tough ally in the battle against mental health challenges. It has been consistently shown to enhance mood, decrease the symptoms of anxiety and depression, and bolster self-esteem and cognitive function.

Physical activity has also been shown to improve sleep quality and reduce feelings of stress, thanks to its ability to regulate neurotransmitters and hormones associated with stress and anxiety, such as cortisol and adrenaline. Furthermore, exercise stimulates the production of endorphins, often referred to as the body's natural mood elevators, which can create feelings of euphoria and general well-being.

For example, running and walking are known to release endorphins, often referred to as "runner's high," which can elevate mood and reduce feelings of anxiety and depression. The psychological benefits extend beyond the biochemical, as these exercises provide a meditative effect, allowing for mental clarity and stress relief. The repetitive motion and focus on breathing create a space for mindfulness, improving overall mental well-being.

For individuals facing the challenges of specific mental health conditions, such as schizophrenia or substance use disorders, exercise offers a complementary therapeutic avenue. By promoting a more active lifestyle, individuals may experience a reduction in psychotic symptoms and an improvement in overall mental health.

Bone and Muscle Health

Exercise is also invaluable for bone and muscle health. Weight-bearing exercises, such as running, help strengthen bones and prevent osteoporosis. Incorporating them into your routine improves muscle strength and endurance, particularly in the lower body, enhancing stability and reducing the risk of falls and injuries later in life.

Reduces the Risks of Neurodegenerative Diseases

The role of exercise also extends into the world of neurodegenerative diseases, where it has been identified as a key factor in reducing the risk of developing conditions like Alzheimer's disease. By enhancing brain-derived neurotrophic factor (BDNF) levels, exercise supports cognitive health and maintains neural plasticity, safeguarding against cognitive decline.

Central to understanding is recognizing its immediate and long-term effects on brain health and cognitive function. Research indicates that physical activity facilitates improved thinking and cognition, not only in the short term but as a protective measure against cognitive decline in later years. This protective effect, coupled with exercise's ability to reduce the risk of developing chronic conditions and enhance mood and sleep quality, presents a convincing case for its inclusion as a key pillar of health.

Enhancing Longevity and Reducing Risk of Early Death

Scientific studies have consistently shown that consistent exercise can reduce the risk of premature death by up to 30% (Warburton, 2006). This remarkable impact on longevity can be attributed to various mechanisms through which physical activity enhances overall health.

Regular exercise helps mitigate risk factors for chronic diseases—such as coronary heart disease, stroke, type II diabetes, and certain cancers—which are major contributors to early mortality globally.

Improved cardiovascular health from regular exercise boosts heart function, lowers blood pressure, and enhances circulation, thereby reducing heart-related disease risks (Kokkinos, 2012). Additionally, physical activity regulates blood sugar levels and improves insulin sensitivity. These effects are crucial for preventing metabolic syndrome and type II diabetes, conditions that can significantly impact life expectancy. Beyond physical health, exercise also benefits mental well-being, further contributing to longevity.

On a cellular level, physical activity has been shown to promote telomere lengthening, associated with aging (Song et al., 2022b). By preserving telomere length, exercise can slow down the aging process, contributing to extended youthfulness and vitality.

Thus, as we navigate the pathways to wellness, the inclusion of regular physical activity emerges as a non-negotiable element of a healthy lifestyle. Its universal applicability, irrespective of age, fitness level, or health status, positions exercise as a versatile and essential practice for all. The challenge, then, is not in recognizing the value of exercise but in integrating this knowledge into daily life, developing routines that accommodate individual preferences, and overcoming the barriers to consistent physical activity.

MY PERSONAL EXPERIENCE WITH EXERCISE

I've observed firsthand the significant impact exercise has had on my physical health, self-perception, and confidence. Integrating regular physical activity into my routine has been instrumental in managing my weight, achieving a consistent and healthy body composition, and enhancing my overall appearance. This transformation has been visible, manifesting in the way I fit into my clothes and carry myself, ultimately boosting my confidence in various aspects of life.

The path to incorporating exercise into my life was gradual and intentional, unfolding alongside my exploration of strategic fasting. Initially, my focus was solely on dietary adjustments, but as I delved deeper into understanding holistic health, I recognized the indispensable role of physical activity. It was not until 2017 that I earnestly began to engage in exercise as a consistent part of my lifestyle.

I started with running, an effective form of physical activity that laid the foundation for my fitness regimen. As I experienced the benefits of running—ranging from improved cardiovascular health to enhanced mental clarity—I was motivated to diversify my exercise routine, including cycling, swimming, and eventually golfing. Each activity added a new layer of challenge and enrichment to my overall fitness journey.

This evolution of my exercise routine was not merely about adding variety; it represented a deeper understanding and appreciation of the synergy between different forms of physical activity and their cumulative benefits on my health. Each new discipline brought unique advantages, contributing to a well-rounded fitness regime that supported my strategic fasting and dietary goals.

Moreover, this journey involved finding synergy between diet and exercise, meticulously learning to balance exercise intensity and frequency with the OMAD approach. It was a gradual and consistent effort that required time, understanding, and patience to avoid overexertion and ensure sustained energy levels throughout the day. This step-by-step approach seamlessly integrated physical activity into my lifestyle, enhancing my dietary strategy and overall well-being.

Below is a detailed exploration of how exercise became a part of my lifestyle.

The Gradual Introduction of Exercise

Running: The Foundation

My genuine commitment to exercise began around 2017, following the establishment of my strategic fasting routine. The weekends became my time to explore the energy and endurance I had built up, leading me to dedicate Saturday mornings to two-hour runs. I followed this routine consistently throughout 2017, laying the groundwork for entering the world of long-distance running. By 2018, the pattern was well established, and I was prepared to challenge myself further by signing up for a marathon, a goal fueled by the miles I had logged and a desire to test my limits.

Participation in Marathon—A Milestone

Participating in that marathon in January 2019 was a key moment in my fitness journey. It was an experience filled with a spectrum of emotions— from joy to pain—that offered me key insights into how my body responded to endurance exercise on the OMAD regimen. It was a learning experience about my body's reaction to long-distance and endurance challenges, particularly within the context of adhering to the OMAD lifestyle.

It was a test of will, where the pain that pushed me to the brink of my physical limits was followed by joy. Despite the struggles, completing the marathon—albeit barely—revealed my body's remarkable adaptability and strength, enriching my understanding of its capabilities through the various phases of my exercise regimen. The lessons learned from this are integral to the narrative I wish to share, detailing the challenges I faced in such a physically demanding event while adhering to OMAD and the readjustments I made in the running distances, ultimately leading me to half marathons.

Cycling: Expanding Horizons

For two years, my focus was primarily on running, cultivating discipline and endurance through countless miles. However, in 2020, my journey took a turn towards cycling, initially integrating short indoor sessions of about 10 to 15 minutes per week into my regimen. Despite these new additions, running remained a cornerstone of my exercise routine, marked by participation in marathons and half marathons.

As the year progressed and the pandemic reshaped our lives, I seized the opportunity to extend cycling outdoors with friends who shared my fitness level. This transition enriched my exercise experience and significantly amplified my cycling efforts—from modest indoor rides to expansive outdoor journeys, clocking in up to 50 to 100 miles weekly. Saturdays became dedicated cycling days, transforming them into hours-long excursions that replaced my usual runs, while Sundays were reserved for lighter runs.

This evolution in my fitness pursuits was not a solo journey. During this period, my wife became my running partner, and we started this running journey together. Her presence matched my skill level and was key to sustaining my motivation. Similarly, as I ventured into cycling, the support and shared enthusiasm of friends who cycled with me kept my spirits high and my pedals turning. This progression from running to embracing cycling fully in 2020 paved the way for an even broader exploration of physical fitness.

Swimming: Enhancing Endurance

In 2021, while maintaining my running and cycling routines, I took up swimming, gradually introducing this new activity to a friend at a similar skill level. We approached swimming with careful progression, incrementally increasing our distances in the pool. This new discipline was added to my regimen without compromising my commitment to running and cycling. I managed to maintain my fitness levels across all activities, ensuring a balanced and comprehensive exercise routine.

Participation in Cypress Sprint Triathlon—Another Milestone

This diversified exercise routine further motivated me to diversify my exercise regimen, leading me to envision triathlons by 2021, a decision fueled by my growing confidence in swimming. So, I participated in the Cypress Sprint Triathlon in July 2021. The event was a significant fitness test, challenging me to integrate running, cycling, and swimming seamlessly. In the Cypress Sprint Triathlon, I steered the course successfully, which included swimming for approximately 500 meters, cycling for about 15 miles, and running a 5k.

This triathlon experience highlighted my commitment to an active lifestyle and marked a key moment in my exercise journey. It represented the fulfillment of my efforts to embrace a multifaceted approach to physical fitness and the continual evolution of my exercise philosophy and its integration into a holistic lifestyle.

I've continued to uphold my active lifestyle, though now in moderation, engaging in running, biking, and swimming just enough to maintain peak condition across these three disciplines. My focus isn't on excessive training but on sustaining an activity that supports my health and well-being.

Golfing: A Leisurely Pursuit

Between 2022 and 2023, I embraced another facet of an active lifestyle by taking up golf. I discovered a community of friends with whom I could share this experience, turning it into both a social activity and a form of exercise. The game allowed me to enjoy leisurely walks across the golf course—each step an exercise in itself—while learning and refining a new skill. This addition highlighted the diversity of my physical activities, contributing to an overall active and balanced lifestyle.

In sharing my journey, I aim to delve deeper into the in-depth understanding I gained about my body and nutrition, particularly during my first full marathon. This experience is crucial to discuss, as it revealed my intense challenges, the moments I nearly gave up, and my body's physical responses under extreme endurance. The reactions of my muscles, the battle with my calves and hamstrings, and the mental strength required to push through are key chapters of my story. These experiences led me to reassess and ultimately adjust the distances in my running regimen and opt for half marathons.

Moreover, there was a process behind finding synergy between my diet and exercise, balancing the intensity and frequency of workouts with the OMAD approach. As we move forward, I want to explore these challenges in greater detail, offering insights into the strength and adaptability required to maintain an active lifestyle within the framework of the OMAD diet.

INTEGRATING PHYSICAL ACTIVITY

As I embarked on my marathon journey, it coincided with a key shift towards cleaner eating and being more mindful about my diet. This period marked a transition into consuming prepackaged salads and rotisserie chicken, selecting the right meals that could align with my newfound dietary consciousness around early 2017.

During this time, weekends became dedicated to physical activity; initially, this involved walking for about an hour on the treadmill each Saturday and Sunday with no other exercise. This routine persisted for approximately three months, with healthy eating accompanying a lot of salads. Then, on the weekends, I gathered the courage and confidence to extend my running outdoors.

Embracing the outdoors marked a significant shift in my journey towards the marathon. Integrating healthy eating habits with my exercise routine, I ventured outside on weekends for two to three hours of walking and running. The convenience of a nearby lake, merely a walking distance from where I lived, provided the perfect circuit for my activities. This lake had a sidewalk that traced a mile-long loop, ideal for setting tangible goals for each session.

I established a routine of walking and jogging around this lake, aiming to complete a set of loops each weekend. Starting with a target of five loops, equivalent to five miles, I gradually increased my ambition to ten loops or ten miles, mixing walking with jogging. This methodical approach to building endurance was about the physical act of running and an integral part of adapting my body and mind to the discipline required for long-distance running. This routine persisted for about a year, laying a solid foundation for my fitness and solidifying my determination to take on a marathon challenge. Witnessing the televised

Houston Marathon made me realize that participating in such an event might be within my reach. This revelation was a turning point, propelling me towards the ambitious goal of completing a marathon, fueled by the consistent effort and dedication I had invested in my weekend exercises by the lake.

By mid-2018, bolstered by my consistent outdoor exercise, I decided to sign up for the marathon. This decision intensified my weekend training to at least three hours on both Saturday and Sunday. Research into marathon preparation emphasized the importance of nutrition, particularly the recommendation of high-sugar sports drinks and energy gels for race day. Given my commitment to mindful eating, I opted against these sugary options, focusing instead on maintaining my diet of vegetables, proteins, and water.

This approach to nutrition, coupled with running in a slightly fasted state, marked a significant phase of my training. I refined my diet further, moving away from prepackaged vegetables to preparing my own meals with healthier carbohydrate sources like sliced potatoes and grilling proteins such as salmon and chicken. This careful attention to nutrition was about sustenance and enhancing my physical performance through better dietary choices.

As the marathon drew closer, my confidence soared, leading me to share my marathon aspirations with family, neighbors, and colleagues. About a month before the event, a milestone 20-mile walk and jog significantly boosted my confidence, reinforcing my belief in the power of my dietary strategy and my body's resilience.

Marathon Milestones: A Test of Limits and Strength

The anticipation built as the marathon day approached. Despite a restless night due to nerves, I woke up feeling energized and ready to face the challenge ahead. The atmosphere at the marathon venue was electrifying, filled with participants buzzing with excitement for the marathon and half marathon events. This energy was precisely what I needed, providing an additional boost to my spirits. Having planned my strategy carefully, including running with music to maintain my morale, I was eager to experience my first race of such scale.

The marathon commenced, and the initial three miles were exhilarating. Powered by adrenaline and the dynamic energy of the crowd, I surged forward with enthusiasm. This initial phase went smoothly, boosted by the upbeat music and the collective energy of the participants. However, as I transitioned from mile six to nine, I noticed a shift in the atmosphere. The marathon runners were now separated from those running the half marathon, leaving fewer people on my path. This change in dynamics made me more conscious of my surroundings and physical state, revealing signs of fatigue I hadn't felt earlier.

At this point, the importance of hydration and nutrition became evident. Approaching the aid station between miles six and nine, I stocked up on energy gels, pocketing five of them, and refreshed myself with water. Interestingly, soon after rehydrating, I craved more water, a sensation that preoccupied my thoughts in the next mile. It was then I remembered the energy gels I had with me. Consuming an energy gel temporarily boosted me, allowing me to pick up my pace slightly. However, this was also when I encountered my first cramp in my right calf, an unexpected challenge I had not experienced in all my training. I adjusted my pace in response, hoping to manage the discomfort and continue the race.

Following that, I became increasingly reliant on the energy gels, consuming a second one in less than half a mile. Despite a brief surge in pace, this led to more cramps in my right and left calf, giving me a new set of challenges. Adjusting my pace offered slight relief, yet the need for both water and more energy gels persisted, particularly between miles six and nine.

A restroom break at mile nine offered a brief respite, yet discomfort remained. Despite consuming additional energy gels, I encountered an insatiable thirst for water—the more I drank, the more I craved, diverging significantly from my usual training regimen. This stage of the race revealed my unexpectedly fast pace, propelled by adrenaline and the race day atmosphere, marking a stark contrast to my training's more measured jog-walk rhythm.

As the marathon progressed towards the 12-mile mark, cramping intensified, now affecting my hamstrings. The transition in my response—from running with music to walking in silence—signaled a shift in strategy aimed at mitigating the discomfort. Interestingly, the cycle of consuming energy gels, experiencing a brief boost followed by increased cramping, persisted, highlighting the complexities of managing energy and pain in real time.

Upon approaching mile 13, the cramps extended to my quads, introducing a new physical challenge I hadn't previously encountered. Every time I felt cramps, I responded by lowering my pace, which temporarily provided relief. But the cramps' persistence clearly revealed the marathon's demands. Reaching the halfmarathon point in two hours and fifteen minutes was a significant milestone.

At this juncture, when a race helper approached and inquired if I wished to quit, offering to escort me directly to the finish line, I was confronted with a choice I hadn't previously considered or expected. His question jolted me, marking the first instance I came across the option of abandoning the challenge. I looked at him and said, "No," and then said to myself, "I have to finish."

I declined because I didn't want to disappoint myself and the circle of family, friends, and colleagues I had confidently informed of my marathon quest. This determination to proceed, despite the option to quit, came from this deep commitment not to let down those aware of my marathon goal. At that point, all I could think about was getting to the next aid station. So I focused on advancing, discovering that walking offered some relief from the debilitating cramps.

Reaching the aid station at mile 14, I had an opportunity for a brief massage and a significant moment to reassess my situation, realizing the disparity between my race day execution and my training regimen. This deviation, propelled by the race's adrenaline, prompted me to abandon the walk-run strategy that had been the cornerstone of my preparation. Instead, I had succumbed to the moment's energy, attempting to run continuously. The decision to walk post-mile 14 emerged as a tactical shift and a moment of introspection and acceptance. It emphasized that the body's output on race day is inextricably linked to the specificity and discipline of one's training.

Despite the urge to resume running, the limitations of my physical condition became apparent, highlighting the fundamental principle that the body can only deliver performance according to its preparation. Thus, walking became my primary mode of progression, a strategy emphasizing consistency between training habits and race day execution.

As I walked, I calculated what it would take to finish the marathon. Determining that 20 minutes per mile would allow me to complete the remaining nine miles within three hours, I set a new goal: to walk and finish the marathon within this timeframe. This period of the race became a significant opportunity for introspection and learning about my body's responses to the varying intensities of physical exertion.

Despite the clarity of the plan, the journey was anything but simple. Periodically, as cramps reduced and energy returned, I felt compelled to jog, only to be met with immediate cramping that forced me to slow down again. This cycle offered valuable insights into the precursors to cramping, teaching me to recognize my body's subtle signals about pacing and endurance. The consumption of energy gels provided a temporary boost, invariably followed by a desire for more energy and more water. I was seemingly caught in a cycle where the relief was short, with an endless desire for more energy boost.

Adjusting my approach due to these physical challenges, my strategy shifted from finishing the race to concentrating on getting to the next aid station, spaced every two miles. Each stop became a checkpoint of rest and recovery, propelling me forward through the most challenging physical challenge I had ever undertaken. The encouragement from spectators, the offers of companionship from fellow runners, and the external validation of my effort were unexpected sources of motivation. They reinforced my resolve, pushing me to persist despite the physical toll.

Approaching mile 23, my understanding of my physical limits and capabilities had heightened significantly. I learned to anticipate the onset of cramps and found ways to mitigate them through minor posture and foot positioning adjustments.

The thought of reaching the finish line carried a weight of expectation of my own and those who had supported me along the way. The anticipation of sharing my story of overcoming and enduring guided me through the final stretches of the race. As the finish line drew nearer, the significance of this moment exceeded personal achievement; it symbolized a shared victory, a collective experience of success despite hardships.

Crossing the finish line was a moment marked by a surge of emotions and the crowd's support, screaming my name and showing encouragement. The sense of accomplishment was overwhelming, contrasting sharply with the immediate thoughts of never wanting to undertake such a challenge again. Even the prospect of participating in a 5k seemed daunting at that moment. However, the sight of the medal and the feelings of relief and pride that followed were incomparable. It represented completing a grueling physical challenge and, above all, a personal victory over my limits.

In the following days, whenever I heard the music that played just before the cramping started, it brought back all the marathon memories. It felt like a true test of my limits and rewarded me in ways I've never experienced before. The sense of achievement wasn't about beating anyone else; it was purely personal, especially significant, given my unique dietary lifestyle. Finishing at the time limit was a victory over my own challenges, not a race against others. This accomplishment, under the constraints of my one-meal-a-day regimen, was incredibly satisfying and pushed me to contemplate my next steps.

In the weeks following the marathon, reflections on this journey prompted a reevaluation of my goals, and I found myself considering another marathon. However, I decided to focus on a half marathon next, curious to see how I could apply the insights gained from my first marathon to a shorter race. This first marathon was just the beginning for me, opening up a new chapter in understanding how I handle different challenges.

Adjusting Running Distances: Impact on Fitness Strategy and Goals

I leveraged the insights gained from my initial marathon to fine-tune my exercise regimen, particularly as I prepared for subsequent half marathons. This strategic shift was about adjusting distances and enhancing my overall fitness strategy.

One of the significant changes post-marathon was the noticeable improvement in my running capability. Where once I had managed a pace of fifteen minutes per mile, I soon found myself running 10Ks at a brisk nine minutes per mile. This leap in performance was evident as I approached the Woodlands half marathon just two months after my full marathon. Armed with experiences from my previous race, I felt more confident and physically prepared.

During this period, I maintained a balanced diet—rich in well-prepared vegetables, grilled proteins, and carefully chosen carbohydrates—which played a crucial role in my performance. I learned to fine-tune my intake of electrolytes, utilizing natural sources like bananas, which proved essential just before running.

Entering the half marathon, I felt robust and eager, driven by a strong start. My energy was high for the initial six miles, and my pace was swift. However, as I progressed, particularly between miles six and nine, I began to experience cramping. This physical setback was a direct result of my initial speed, which, while exhilarating, proved to be too aggressive. This experience emphasized the importance of managing my pace more cautiously. By moderating my speed, I was able to reduce the occurrence of cramps, allowing for a more consistent pace throughout the race.

Additionally, I refined my hydration and nutrition strategy. Instead of relying on energy gels, which had previously exacerbated my muscle cramps, I focused on maintaining hydration with water alone. This adjustment was crucial between miles nine and twelve, where my sole focus was managing my body's response to the exertion.

This strategic shift proved instrumental in the subsequent races, providing vital insights into my body's responses and helping me further tailor my approach. Each half marathon offered new data points on my physical responses and allowed me to refine my strategy further. It became a testing ground for these new strategies, enabling me to understand better the balance between speed, hydration, and endurance.

Ultimately, this led to a significant decision: to continue enjoying half marathons while optimizing my race day strategies to align with my body's needs. The combination of intense weekend training, a meticulously planned diet, and careful race-day nutrition allowed me to perform optimally at this distance while minimizing the physical challenges associated with full marathons. By the time I participated in another race in October, I had honed my method to rely solely on water. This approach helped me manage my physical responses better and improved my race performance significantly.

Thus, my decision marked a significant turning point in my fitness journey, affirming my commitment to mastering the half marathon as my preferred race format. Concentrating on half marathons, I could continue challenging myself while maintaining a balance supporting my well-being and daily life.

Continuing my journey, the next significant race was a half marathon in October, which differed considerably from the one I ran in March. For this race, I strictly used water to manage my hydration; notably, my pace had improved significantly. This race highlighted my ability to control cramping through pace management; I experienced it only once, around mile 11, due to a significant increase in my speed.

Despite this, I managed the cramp by reducing my speed, much like my previous strategies had taught me. Notably, while I limited myself to drinking water just once during the race, it highlighted a recurring need—whenever I drank, I felt the need for more. This realization was a turning point; I felt confident I had mastered the nuances of running a half marathon.

Motivated by my improvements and insights, I revisited the idea of running another full marathon to test how my body would react to these refined strategies. In January 2020, I participated in my second marathon. The first half went exceptionally well; I managed to maintain a good pace with minimal intake of fluids or energy gels and experienced little to no cramping. However, the latter half of the race revealed a critical need for nutrition to sustain my energy levels, leading me to alternate between walking and jogging. This experience reaffirmed my decision that half marathons were more conducive to my lifestyle, dietary habits, and training routines.

Reflecting on my training, it's important to note that my regimen was consistent: I dedicated my weekends to intensive training sessions of two to three hours and reserved weekdays for rest and light walks. This routine had formed the foundation of my preparation for over a year and a half. After completing my second full marathon, I resolved to focus solely on half marathons. This choice was about adjusting to physical demands and aligning my sporting endeavors with my overall lifestyle and dietary habits, allowing for a sustainable balance that enhanced my well-being without the extreme physical toll of longer distances.

5

BALANCING OMAD DIET AND EXERCISE

Finding synergy between my diet and exercise routines has been a progressive and enlightening journey. Initially, my focus was predominantly on running, which I supported nutritionally through two distinct phases.

I relied on prepackaged vegetables paired with rotisserie chicken—a practical approach that supported my early running days from 2017 through the early months of 2020. As I progressed, this evolved into a regimen of carefully prepared vegetables and grilled proteins—primarily chicken—which became the staples of my diet as I maintained my focus on running.

The first quarter of 2020 marked a key shift in my routine, where I began incorporating cycling into my regimen. Starting with modest sessions, approximately an hour each week, I quickly discovered a growing passion for cycling. This addition coincided with the onset of the pandemic in March 2020, which altered my daily structure significantly. Working from home intensified my exercise schedule; I seized this opportunity to cycle for an hour during my lunch breaks on alternate days while maintaining near-daily runs.

In June, I transitioned my cycling from indoor to outdoor settings. Instead of the confined one-hour indoor sessions, I expanded my cycling activities in the open park environment on alternate days. This provided a refreshing change of scenery and allowed me to engage more dynamically with the environment, enhancing both the enjoyment and effectiveness of my workouts.

I also adjusted the structure of my weekly routine; Sundays were designated as complete rest days to allow for adequate recovery. The remaining days were split between running and cycling, ensuring that I was consistently active while listening to my body's needs and responses. This new rhythm diversified my physical activities and expanded the window for nutritional experimentation.

As my physical activities increased and my exercise routines became more rigorous with running and cycling, I realized the necessity of adapting my diet to support my increased activity levels. This led to another dietary shift from the grilled chicken and vegetable-based diet towards incorporating a wider variety of proteins. Seafood became a predominant component of my meals, with shrimp, fish, and occasionally scallops enriching my nutrient intake. Alongside these, I enjoyed various vegetables, such as eggplant, spinach, bell peppers, cauliflower, and broccoli. My preparation method also evolved; I began to cook and stir-fry the potatoes, enhancing my meals' flavor and nutritional value.

By mid-2021, my curiosity about fitness enhancement led me to transition to a vegetarian diet to support my cycling and running endeavors. The vegetarian diet included a mix of lentils, chickpeas, and occasionally black-eyed peas enriched with robust spices. Complementing these proteins were carbohydrates like sweet potatoes and nutritious additions such as egg whites and spinach, often accompanied by avocados, which provided healthy fats.

The impact of these dietary adjustments on my physical performance was substantial. By October 2021, I had not only adapted fully to the vegetarian diet but had also reached new heights in my athletic performance, achieving personal records (PRs) in both cycling and half marathons. This period of intensive physical activity, paired with a nutrient-rich vegetarian diet, enhanced my performance by up to 10%, proving that there can be a powerful combination of tailored nutrition and dedicated training.

Additionally, in 2021, I began incorporating swimming into my routine, which added variety and prepared me for a new challenge—triathlons. My approach to swimming was gradual; starting about three months before a triathlon event in July, I trained consistently, alternating days to build endurance. Initially aiming to swim 300 to 500 meters per session, I noticed steady improvement.

However, despite these successes, I recognized the need for further dietary adjustments to meet new physical goals since I observed a decrease in muscle mass. This observation led me to contemplate enhancements to my diet to increase muscle definition and overall energy levels, which are crucial for my athletic pursuits and my professional and daily activities. This ongoing adjustment process highlights the dynamic nature of finding the right balance between diet and exercise, where changes in one aspect necessitate thoughtful modifications in the other to achieve a harmonious and effective synergy.

Continuing my journey into 2022, I transitioned back to a more balanced diet, a shift that aligned with a refined understanding of my fitness goals and priorities. At this stage, my objectives were clearly defined: I sought to maintain mental clarity and high performance in my professional life while ensuring that I could still participate and enjoy half marathons, swimming, and cycling events without the pressure of breaking previous records. My motivations had evolved; I was no longer driven by the ambition to achieve a seven-minute mile running pace, swim at a pace of two minutes per hundred meters, or maintain 20+ mph cycling speeds but was focused on sustaining an active lifestyle that brought me joy and fulfillment.

This phase of my fitness journey highlighted the importance of flexibility and attentiveness to dietary and exercise regimes, highlighting how adaptive strategies are essential for sustaining long-term health and fitness goals.

OPTIMIZING HEALTH BENEFITS WITH PHYSICAL ACTIVITY IN THE OMAD LIFESTYLE

Thus, integrating physical activity with the OMAD lifestyle and finding the right balance necessitates a keen understanding of one's physical capabilities and limits. By a certain point in my journey, my focused training in half marathons and cycling had sharpened my understanding of my optimal performance speeds and physical limits, essential for preventing overexertion and ensuring steady progress in shorter distances. A disciplined approach to nutrition played a key role in supporting this active lifestyle. My dietary regime was stringent; I eliminated all sugary drinks, including sodas and commercially available sports drinks, often laden with sugars. I restricted fluids in my diet to water, coffee, and occasionally herbal teas—choices that supported hydration without compromising my health goals.

Adhering strictly to the OMAD principle, I consumed my single daily meal only after completing my workouts, regardless of their intensity. This practice ensured that my body was refueled effectively for recovery and the next day's activities. My meals, prepared post-exercise, were substantial enough to satisfy my nutritional needs until the following day. This strategy supported my physical exertion through a well-timed and nutritious meal. It maintained the discipline required to benefit from the OMAD lifestyle without succumbing to overeating or nutritional imbalance.

Through this meticulous blend of disciplined eating, careful monitoring of physical exertion, and strategic meal timing, I could optimize the health benefits of my activities while ensuring that I did not push my body beyond its recuperative capabilities. This approach highlights the importance of understanding and listening to one's body, especially when balancing intense physical activity with dietary practices like OMAD.

EXERCISE PLANS

Creating Customizable Exercise Routines

Reflecting on the development of adaptable exercise routines, the process hinges on recognizing and building upon foundational fitness principles and individual progression. My journey into fitness started with running, an activity I approached as an absolute beginner. Initially, I incorporated simple walking into my routine, a straightforward, low-intensity exercise that anyone can start with, regardless of their fitness level.

Thanks to a diet rich in vegetables and lean proteins, I began to see sustained improvements in mental clarity and work performance. My walking gradually evolved into jogging and eventually into consistent running. This progression highlights the importance of allowing the body to adapt to increased physical demands gradually. Over time, as my endurance and strength developed, I was able to tackle more challenging goals, such as running marathons and later focusing on half marathons, illustrating a natural progression from basic to more demanding physical activities.

I integrated cycling into my routine following a similar incremental approach at very low intensities, which is an excellent starting point for beginners. As my comfort with cycling grew, I increased the intensity and began cycling in a park with peers of similar skill levels. This social aspect of exercising can be highly motivating and provides a benchmark for measuring personal improvement. Eventually, as my skills and confidence grew, I started cycling with more seasoned professionals, which pushed my limits and enhanced my performance.

The essence of building an exercise routine is maintaining consistency and gradually increasing the challenge. For beginners, starting with low-intensity activities like walking or light cycling and gradually increasing the duration and intensity can be a practical approach. For intermediate enthusiasts, incorporating varied terrains and longer distances can provide the necessary challenge. Advanced individuals might focus on refining their techniques and increasing speed or resistance, pushing towards more professional goals like races or marathons.

Fundamentally, every exercise routine should begin with achievable goals and gradually build up in complexity and intensity. This approach helps maintain a steady improvement curve and ensures that the body is not overexerted, allowing for sustained progress. Each step of the routine, whether it's for a beginner or an experienced athlete, should be tailored to individual needs, current fitness levels, and long-term objectives, ensuring that each routine is both challenging and rewarding.

6

OVERCOMING CHALLENGES

Transitioning into a One-Meal-A-Day (OMAD) lifestyle presents unique challenges that test physical endurance and mental resilience since it involves a significant shift in dietary habits, social areas, and psychological domains. Moreover, it requires understanding and overcoming various obstacles that can affect anyone attempting this significant change in their daily routine.

Initially, the adjustment to OMAD can be daunting due to the natural occurrence of hunger pangs and the social pressures of dining conventions. The key to overcoming these early challenges lies in distinguishing between true hunger and habitual eating patterns. This realization often stems from witnessing the immediate benefits, which provide the motivation needed to sustain any lifestyle change. As individuals adapt to OMAD, they learn to manage their hunger and strategically choose environments that support their dietary choices.

Moreover, maintaining motivation amid a lifestyle that contrasts with conventional dietary norms requires robust strategies. Structuring meals meticulously during the workweek, allowing for flexibility on weekends, and aligning meal timing with physical activity levels are all crucial. These practices help sustain physical energy and ensure one's social and familial life remains enriched and stress-free. Through this chapter, I will delve into the challenges I faced transitioning to the OMAD lifestyle and the strategies that helped me overcome those challenges. The purpose is to offer insights into how one can successfully live with OMAD amidst various challenges, ensuring a balanced approach supporting health and personal fulfillment.

COMMON CHALLENGES AND SOLUTIONS: ADJUSTMENT PERIOD DIFFICULTIES

1. Managing Hunger Pangs

One of the first and most significant challenges I encountered when I began the OMAD lifestyle was managing the hunger pangs that inevitably came with delaying my meals. Initially, distinguishing between true hunger and habitual eating patterns was not straightforward. Over time, however, I began to recognize my body's signals, which were often more about habit than actual hunger.

Adopted Solutions

Identifying Hunger vs. Habit

To overcome this challenge, I focused on the benefits that delaying meals brought to my life, such as enhanced mental clarity, increased focus, and a boost in creativity. These improvements were motivational and instrumental in helping me adhere to the OMAD schedule. Whenever I experienced hunger pangs, I reminded myself of these benefits, reinforcing the reason behind my choice to adopt this eating pattern. This mental strategy was crucial in navigating through the initial adjustment phase and maintaining my commitment to the OMAD lifestyle.

Meal Timing Adjustments and Mindful Consumption Practices

Moreover, I discovered effective methods to overcome this challenge by experimenting with meal timing and integrating mindful consumption practices like drinking black coffee or sipping water throughout the day to curb appetite. These adjustments allowed me to maintain concentration and productivity, emphasizing the adaptability required to embrace the OMAD lifestyle successfully.

I found that incorporating black coffee into my routine was an effective strategy for curbing hunger. Initially, I wasn't a fan of coffee without sweeteners, but its benefits in suppressing appetite and enhancing concentration were significant. On days I chose to reduce my coffee intake, I would sip water throughout the day to manage hunger.

This simple change noticeably improved my concentration and ability to absorb and engage with complex information, helping me at my work. Realizing my dietary habits were crucial to achieving peak performance, the positive impact of meal timing became my catalyst for a more deliberate approach to eating. Introducing delays in my meal schedule sharpened my focus and allowed me to fulfill my responsibilities with greater efficacy. Coupled with the benefits of black coffee, which further aided my concentration and hunger management, I incorporated this adjustment into my daily routine, enhancing my professional engagement and overall productivity.

This methodical approach played a key role in managing hunger pangs. It emphasized the importance of listening to my body and responding with mindful choices, whether leveraging the appetite-suppressing properties of black coffee or hydrating with water to stave off hunger. Embracing these strategies facilitated a smoother transition into OMAD.

2. Lack of Guidance and Supportive Environment

Embarking on the One-Meal-A-Day lifestyle brought another challenge: the absence of mentorship or guidance. Initially, I found myself navigating without a guide or mentor to help me understand how to effectively delay my meals while keeping my health in optimal condition. There were few accessible role models or proven frameworks that aligned with this unconventional approach. Delaying meals, optimizing nutrition, and maintaining health through this regimen required me to rely heavily on self-education.

Adopted Solutions

Self-Guided Learning and Validation through Experience

To overcome this obstacle, I committed myself to an intensive period of self-guided learning. This involved extensive reading on nutrition, intermittent fasting, and the physiological impacts of meal timing. More critically, I embraced a trial-and-error method by experimenting with various dietary compositions and observing their effects on my body and performance. Each race I participated in served as a live experiment to test the effectiveness of my dietary choices.

As I completed more races and continued to adjust my eating window and meal content, the positive changes in my performance and well-being began to solidify my confidence in OMAD. This hands-on approach allowed me to gradually build a robust understanding of balancing my nutritional intake effectively within one meal per day, ensuring I had enough energy to meet my physical and professional demands.

Verification of OMAD Benefits

The ultimate confirmation of the OMAD lifestyle's benefits came from the noticeable improvements in my race times and overall fitness. These successes provided the concrete evidence needed to validate my self-developed eating strategy. Over time, as my achievements became more visible, they served as personal reassurances and persuasive testimonials I could share with friends, family, and fellow athletes. This experience highlighted the importance of patience, personal exploration, and the value of learning from one's experiences to adapt to and thrive within the OMAD lifestyle.

3. Monotony in Prepackaged Meals

As I integrated the OMAD lifestyle with an exercise routine, I initially opted for prepackaged meals to simplify my diet. These convenient meals supported my goals of maintaining mental clarity and a lean physique. However, after some time, it became boring. The repetitive nature of consuming the same types of vegetables and proteins day after day became uninspiring, posing a risk to my commitment to the OMAD lifestyle.

Adopted Solutions

Diversifying Meal Options

To address the boredom associated with my dietary routine, I diversified my meal options. I explored various brands and types of prepackaged vegetables that offered multiple choices. Through experimentation, I developed five distinct kinds of salads, each with unique flavors and dressings. These included a kale-based salad, a cabbage-focused option, and a lettuce-based salad, each paired with dressings that ranged from fruity poppy seed with peach to a spicy Chipotle and an exotic ginger flavor.

Strategy for Weekend Flexibility

Additionally, I allowed myself more flexibility on weekends. This approach enabled me to enjoy a variety of meals and cater to my nutritional needs, especially after intensive workouts. By blending these prepackaged salads with rotisserie chicken, I created quick meals rich in nutrients and satisfying. This method effectively countered the monotony of my diet and reaffirmed my commitment to maintaining a healthy lifestyle through OMAD and regular exercise.

This strategy of embracing flexibility on weekends has also been one of the most effective in maintaining my motivation and commitment to the OMAD lifestyle. It centered heavily on structuring my eating habits during the workweek. Monday through Friday provided a framework where I could rigorously adhere to my meal timing, experiencing firsthand the benefits of such discipline, facilitating consistency in my dietary choices, and reinforcing the positive impacts of delayed eating.

On weekends, I aligned this with time spent on social activities and family engagements. This adaptation was not merely about enjoying a varied diet but also strategically choosing recovery meals that supported the increased physical activity of my weekend exercise routines. Doing so ensured that the more relaxed weekend eating did not compromise the gains achieved during the structured weekdays.

4. Managing Recovery Meals and Weight Fluctuation

Integrating exercise into my OMAD lifestyle presented a unique set of challenges, particularly around managing recovery meals. As my physical activity increased, particularly on weekends, I noticed a direct correlation between feeling tired post-exercise and experiencing increased hunger. This posed a significant challenge in balancing my meal intake to effectively recover without compromising my weight management goals. Initially, I observed fluctuations in my weight, which needed careful handling to maintain a steady weight that supported both my dietary and fitness objectives.

Adopted Solutions

Strategic Planning of Recovery Meals

To address this issue, I meticulously planned my recovery meals to ensure they were satisfying and nutritionally balanced. Recognizing the importance of meal composition and timing, I focused on including a mix of macronutrients to replenish energy stores and aid muscle recovery without leading to excessive caloric intake. My recovery meals typically included a higher proportion of proteins and complex carbohydrates, which helped stabilize my energy levels and mitigate the post-exercise hunger spikes.

Adapting Meal Content Based on Activity Level

Additionally, I tailored my weekend meals to align with my increased physical activity. This involved enhancing the nutritional density of my meals during more active days to accommodate higher energy expenditure. By adjusting the quantity and quality of foods consumed on these days, particularly increasing vegetable intake and incorporating lean proteins, I was able to maintain a balanced weight and improve my overall recovery times.

This sustainable approach to managing my recovery meals helped stabilize my weight and enhanced my performance in both routine exercise and competitive events. It became clear that adequate recovery nutrition was crucial for maintaining the long-term sustainability of combining intense exercise with the OMAD diet.

5. Navigating Social Dining While Maintaining an OMAD Lifestyle

Integrating the OMAD lifestyle into my social life posed a distinct challenge, particularly when dining with family, colleagues, and friends. During the initial stages, while I had embraced this new eating pattern with enthusiasm due to its clear benefits on my mental clarity and weight, extending this practice into social settings required careful navigation. Divergent dietary preferences within my social circles and frequent social gatherings posed a risk of derailing my dietary regimen.

Adopted Solutions

Strategic Food Choices and Communication

To manage this challenge effectively, I adopted a proactive approach in various social dining scenarios. With my family, I maintained my dietary choices during our meals together while allowing them the flexibility to eat as they preferred. This approach demonstrated the effectiveness of my diet and gradually influenced their eating habits without imposing restrictions.

I want to share one particularly challenging moment during my first family vacation after adopting this new eating pattern. Vacations had always been a time for relaxation and less dietary restraint. However, recognizing the need to maintain my lifestyle, I sought vacation destinations that supported my health goals. These places needed to have good running trails, access to gyms, or proximity to grocery stores that offered healthy options.

Instead of viewing these requirements as limitations, I embraced them as opportunities to enhance my vacation experience. Each morning began with physical activity—running, jogging, or walking—setting a positive tone for the day and aligning with my OMAD principles. This activity boosted my physical health and enhanced my mental clarity and overall enjoyment of the vacation.

By carefully balancing the flexibility in my diet with structured physical activities, I could continue enjoying my vacations without deviating from my health goals. Integrating these elements allowed me to maintain energy levels and mental alertness, converting what could have been a challenge into a refreshing component of my holiday routine. This approach ensured that even while on vacation, I could sustain the lifestyle that had become so beneficial, affirming that the joy derived from this lifestyle could seamlessly extend into all areas of my life.

In professional settings with colleagues, where lunches and work-related gatherings were common, I steered the group towards restaurants that offered healthy, diverse options aligned with my dietary needs. I identified three specific restaurants known for their healthy menus, ensuring I could stick to my OMAD principles without feeling socially isolated. These venues became regular spots supporting my dietary goals and social interactions.

Adapting to Social Gatherings with Personalized Contributions

Furthermore, in more informal settings with friends or neighbors, I would bring my own prepared dishes to gatherings. This ensured I had suitable food options and introduced my peers to healthier alternatives, subtly advocating for the nutritional benefits of my choices. By bringing items such as trays of fruits and specially prepared snacks, I managed to enjoy social occasions without compromising my diet.

These strategies significantly eased the integration of OMAD into my daily life, making it feasible to maintain this lifestyle consistently, regardless of the social context. They also minimized the dietary divergence in social settings, helping me avoid potential setbacks while fostering a supportive environment around my dietary choices.

6. Nutritional Adequacy During Intensified Exercise

As the pandemic unfolded, I engaged in more rigorous and frequent exercise routines, including extended cycling sessions and longer running periods. This increase in physical activity highlighted a significant challenge: the nutritional insufficiency of my existing diet, which primarily consisted of vegetables and rotisserie chicken. It became apparent that this diet was inadequate for sustaining the higher energy demands of my intensified exercise regimen.

Adopted Solutions

Tailored Nutrition for Enhanced Athletic Performance

To address this challenge, I embarked on a meticulous dietary experimentation and research journey to understand the optimal balance of proteins, carbohydrates, fats, and hydration necessary to support not just any lifestyle but one marked by vigorous physical activity. This exploration led me to reconsider and eventually move away from common athletic supplements like sugary energy drinks and gels, which did not align with my health objectives.

Adopting a Wholesome, Customized Diet

Instead, I opted for natural alternatives that complemented my health goals. I incorporated homemade preparations, utilizing natural sweeteners like dates to enhance my meals without compromising on nutritional integrity. My focus shifted towards a more plant-based diet, initially integrating more seafood before fully transitioning to a vegetarian diet rich in lentils, chickpeas, and other protein-rich legumes.

This dietary shift proved key in aligning with my health perspectives and significantly boosting my athletic performance.

By carefully selecting and preparing my meals, I could sustain longer training sessions and recover more effectively, allowing me to maintain—and even lose—weight while improving my cycling and running. This was particularly evident in my ability to handle distances up to 60 miles on the bike and complete halfmarathons more effectively.

7. Adjusting Diet for Muscle Gain

As I progressed in my fitness journey, a new challenge emerged: the desire to enhance my muscle mass for better performance and aesthetics. This goal led me back to incorporating a mixed diet, reintroducing animal proteins after a period focused on plant-based sources.

Adopted Solutions

Reintroduction and Adaptation to Animal Proteins

Transitioning back to a diet that included animal proteins was not straightforward. My body initially resisted this change, unaccustomed as it had become to digesting meat after an extended period of vegetarianism. The adjustment phase involved careful reintroduction and monitoring how different proteins affected my body, requiring patience and persistence.

Over time, my body adapted, allowing me to gain the muscle mass I aimed for effectively. Although challenging, this dietary shift ultimately enabled me to enhance my physical strength and improve my performance in various activities.

8. Communicating the OMAD Lifestyle and Fitness Strategy

As I progressed and the results of my OMAD lifestyle became visibly apparent—marked improvements in physique and enhanced vitality—questions arose from colleagues, friends, and family. They noticed the significant changes, from my increased fitness to my leaner appearance, and were curious about the methods behind my transformation.

Adapted Solutions

Educating and Demonstrating Through Personal Experience

The primary challenge was articulating the benefits and practicalities of the OMAD lifestyle and its integration with a rigorous fitness regimen. Initially, I found it difficult to convey the dietary aspects effectively, particularly how to balance meal timing, content, and the overall nutritional strategy that supported my physical activities.

While I could share my experiences and the physical training aspects—such as progressing from walking to running and preparing for half marathons—explaining the nutritional foundation essential for such endurance activities was more challenging. The complexity of defining the synchronization of meal timing with energy requirements and recovery needs meant that I often fell short in communicating the full scope of the lifestyle's benefits and requirements.

Over time, as I participated in more races and my lifestyle choices consistently showed positive results, I developed better ways to share both the fitness and nutritional aspects of my journey. By focusing initially on the physical elements, which were easier for people to relate to and implement, I gradually introduced the more complex nutritional strategies as their interest and readiness to adapt increased.

REFLECTIONS ON ACHIEVEMENTS AND CONTINUOUS IMPROVEMENT

Reflecting on my journey with the OMAD lifestyle, I consider my day-to-day routine one of my greatest achievements. From hydrating upon waking to maintaining a rigorous exercise regimen and excelling in my professional life, each element is proof of the disciplined lifestyle I've crafted. This routine enables me to participate in demanding physical activities, such as running a half marathon monthly or engaging in 50-mile cycling sessions, reinforcing my physical strength and mental clarity.

Over time, what began as a concerted effort has seamlessly transitioned into habit. This evolution in my lifestyle is particularly evident in how I manage my diet and exercise. Selecting and preparing meals that support my active lifestyle has become intuitive, allowing me to nourish my body efficiently without the need to count calories meticulously. My body's natural cues now guide my eating and exercise intensity, indicating when I have reached satiety or need to adjust my pace during runs.

Despite these successes, I remain committed to continuous self-improvement. Optimizing my health and fitness continues as I seek to advance to the next stages of wellness and mindfulness, aiming for deeper self-actualization. This ongoing process enhances my well-being and strengthens the connections within my social and professional circles, surrounded by those who share similar health and fitness goals.

7

DOCUMENTING THE JOURNEY

KEEPING A JOURNAL

The Power of Written Reflection

Documenting the journey through detailed journaling has been a transformative practice in my commitment to the one-meal-a-day (OMAD) lifestyle. By meticulously recording daily dietary habits and emotional states, I have gained meaningful insights into how specific foods impact my energy levels, mood, and overall health. This practice of written reflection has enhanced my self-awareness and solidified my dedication to maintaining a balanced and nutritious diet.

Initially, journaling helped me quantify and understand my meals' nutritional content. For instance, by documenting, I realized that my typical meal comprised an appropriate balance of proteins, carbohydrates, and fats, totaling about 2,500 calories—adequate to sustain both my metabolism and physical activities. This revelation was crucial in ensuring that each meal was nutritionally complete, effectively supporting both my physical exercises and cognitive functions.

Later on, my journaling practice evolved into a habit. After consistently documenting my diet and exercise for over a year and a half, the process became instinctual. I reached a point where I no longer needed to write down every detail; I had internalized the rhythms and requirements of my dietary and exercise routine. This intuitive knowledge enabled me to effortlessly plan my grocery shopping and meals well in advance—up to a month or two—without needing to consult written notes. This transition from documented planning to mental mapping emphasized how habitual the process of maintaining my OMAD lifestyle had become.

One significant aspect of documenting my journey was the ability to set and surpass daily fitness and dietary goals. Each journal entry acted as a record of the previous day's activities, allowing me to evaluate my performance and set incremental goals. For instance, if one day's activity involved a 20-minute walk or cycle, simply extending this duration by a minute the following day marked a personal achievement. This process of continuous improvement was not limited to exercise but extended to dietary habits as well.

By noting down details such as occasional indulgence in less healthy options like chips, I could strategically plan substitutions for the next day that better align with my health objectives. The act of writing simplified complex dietary and fitness regimes into a visible, manageable format, making it easier to adjust behaviors and maintain progress toward my overall health goals. This straightforward method of reflection and planning ensured that each day was a step in the right direction and a conscious advancement towards a healthier lifestyle, reinforcing the benefits and motivations of the OMAD journey.

JOURNALING TECHNIQUES

Structuring for Clarity and Motivation

The initial motivation for my meticulous journaling stemmed from a significant increase in my physical activities around the onset of the pandemic. Engaging in more frequent cycling and running necessitated a corresponding augmentation in my nutritional intake. This period led me to experiment with a variety of foods available at the grocery store, from different types of vegetables and meats to carbohydrates and herbs like turmeric and ginger.

Journaling became a tool for immediate feedback on the effects of these dietary experiments on my body. For instance, after incorporating ginger into my post-workout recovery, I noted a marked improvement in muscle relaxation and recovery speed. Conversely, consuming minty tea in the morning made me feel relaxed but slightly sleepy, prompting me to reserve it for evening consumption to better align with my body's natural rhythm.

This daily documentation of both my diet and exercise allowed me to adjust my food intake in real time based on the physical demands and responses. It also helped me monitor potential health symptoms amid pandemic concerns. Fortunately, I never got sick throughout that period. Recording these details fostered a deeper understanding of how specific foods influenced my mood and energy levels, enabling me to make informed adjustments to optimize my overall well-being.

Most Effective Journaling Technique

The most effective journaling technique I've adopted is using a pen and notebook, one of the most straightforward and manageable processes. Each evening or the following morning, I document my daily intake and activities. This routine takes about 10 minutes, reflecting the simplicity of the approach.

After several months, this handwritten journal can be transferred to a digital format, allowing for easier tracking and pattern recognition. Often, I find that many entries are repetitive, indicating consistent habits or routines that either reinforce my lifestyle goals or highlight areas needing change. This digital transition further simplifies the process, making it more efficient and providing a long-term overview of my progress and habits.

My journal layout involved splitting entries into two primary sections: one for nutrition and the other for workouts. The nutrition column is meticulously detailed, capturing every meal and snack to track dietary habits comprehensively. The exercise column is straightforward, where I might note "20-minute run" or "20-minute walk."

This simple yet effective structure allowed me to track the variety of foods consumed—from proteins to carbohydrates and fats—and the corresponding impact on my body during workouts. Maintaining this record consistently Monday through Friday, with some flexibility on weekends, allowed me to capture a complete picture of my dietary habits and physical activities without becoming a burden.

Over time, this simple act of daily documentation has evolved into a habit, providing immediate insights and enabling quick adjustments based on my body's feedback. Utilizing apps to track specific nutritional data helped me align my intake with recommended dietary standards, affirming the adequacy of my meal compositions in a scientifically verifiable manner.

Regular journaling could transition one's dietary awareness from a conscious effort to an automatic routine, greatly simplifying the process of meal planning and grocery shopping. Now, I can mentally plan meals for extended periods without needing to refer to written notes, yet adhere closely to the nutritional balance established through my earlier journaling efforts.

TROUBLESHOOTING DIETARY AND EXERCISE CHALLENGES WITH JOURNALING

Journaling has proven invaluable in addressing and overcoming specific challenges related to diet and exercise. One significant advantage has been the ability to troubleshoot issues that arise during intensive training periods or dietary shifts.

For instance, I meticulously recorded my dietary intake and exercise routines leading up to a major race while on a vegetarian diet. It provided crucial insights when I achieved my best time in a half marathon. Post-race, I could analyze the data to understand the effects of different aspects of my training. An example of this was identifying knee discomfort during races, which I traced back to an imbalance in my training focus. My journal revealed that my preparations had overly concentrated on uphill training, neglecting the impact of downhill running. Recognizing this, I adjusted my training to include more downhill exercises, alleviating knee pain and improving my race performance.

Furthermore, the journal helped me fine-tune my diet to support my recovery and performance. For example, noting the beneficial effects of ginger, whether as a tea or included in meals, helped me understand its role in muscle recovery.

Similarly, I observed that incorporating specific vegetables like spinach enhanced my endurance and overall well-being during races. These observations allowed me to make informed decisions about which foods to emphasize or eliminate from my diet to optimize my health and athletic performance.

By systematically documenting each element of my diet and exercise, I could make immediate corrections based on how my body responded, leading to tangible improvements in both my physical health and race outcomes. This systematic approach to journaling facilitated a deeper understanding of my body's needs and highlighted the effectiveness of adapting my lifestyle in real time based on documented experiences and results.

Here are a few tables recreated from my journal showcasing how I documented my exercise routines and dietary habits. These entries provide an in-depth look at my daily regimen, capturing my journey toward improved health and performance. Through these records, I could track progress, identify patterns, and make necessary adjustments to optimize my training and nutrition strategies.

Daily Meal Composition & Workout - Monday, 2/7/2022			
Beverages	**Protein, Carbs, Fat, Fruits & Vegetables**	**Snacks**	**Workout**
Coffee	Quinoa, Plantains, Avocados	Almonds	Run (outdoors)
Water	Bananas, Carrots, Cauliflower, Broccoli	Trail Mix	31 mins; 4.1 miles; 7:39 min/mile

Daily Meal Composition & Workout - Tuesday, 2/8/2022

Beverages	Protein, Carbs, Fat, Fruits & Vegetables	Snacks	Workout
Coffee	Eggs, Sweet Potatoes, Avocados	Almonds	Bike (Indoors)
Water	Strawberries, Spinach, Bell Peppers, Tomatoes	Trail Mix	16 mins; 6.21 miles; 22.5mph

Daily Meal Composition & Workout - Wednesday, 2/9/2022

Beverages	Protein, Carbs, Fat, Fruits & Vegetables	Snacks	Workout
Coffee	Peas, Potatoes, Avocados	Brownies	Run (Outdoors)
Water	Pears, Cauliflower, Broccoli		17 mins; 2.4 miles; 7:13 min/mile

These first three tables from 2022 from my journal illustrate how I meticulously documented my diet and exercise routines leading up to key events.

Daily Meal Composition & Workout - Monday, 2/5/2024

Beverages	Protein, Carbs, Fat, Fruits & Vegetables	Snacks	Workout
Coffee	Beef, Russet Potatoes, Avocados	Dark Chocolate	Treadmill Workout. 12.5% Incline.
Water	Apples, Cauliflower, Broccoli	Mixed Nuts	30 mins; 4.0 mph

Daily Meal Composition & Workout - Tuesday, 2/6/2024

Beverages	Protein, Carbs, Fat, Fruits & Vegetables	Snacks	Workout
Coffee	Shrimp, Sweet Potatoes, Avocados	Dark Chocolate	Bike (Indoors)
Water	Peach, Squash	Trail Mix	30 mins; Zone 2 workout

Daily Meal Composition & Workout - Wednesday, 2/7/2024			
Beverages	**Protein, Carbs, Fat, Fruits & Vegetables**	**Snacks**	**Workout**
Coffee	Chicken, Petit Potatoes, Avocados	Dark Chocolate	Base strength workout - Pull-ups,
Water	Oranges, Eggplant, Broccoli		Chin-ups, Crunches, Push-ups – 30mins

The above three tables show a detailed journal entry documenting my diet and exercise regimen over several days in 2024. The journal is divided into daily segments, each starting with the date, followed by a list of consumed food and drinks and the specifics of my workouts. This journaling reflects my methodical approach to preparing for my races and triathlons, capturing daily habits contributing to my performance.

This level of detail continues each day, highlighting the specific foods and beverages consumed and the types and durations of exercise, including running and cycling. By logging meals and workouts, you can ensure a structured routine that supports your athletic goals.

REFLECTIVE LEARNING: INSIGHTS AND REALIZATIONS

Reflecting on the journey of maintaining a detailed journal, one of the key realizations I've come to appreciate is the intrinsic value of the very act of writing down daily activities related to fitness and nutrition. The process itself, beginning from the first entry, represents a significant milestone. This initial step of documenting one's daily regime marks the start of a committed path toward health and well-being.

The insight here is that the journey toward self-improvement and understanding one's dietary and physical activity patterns begins with that first logged entry. Each recorded detail, no matter how minor it may seem at the time, contributes to a larger narrative of personal growth and development. This documentation concretely affirms one's dedication to the health goals, providing a tangible record of progress and challenges.

From a broader perspective, these journal entries are the foundational steps that inspire further achievements, such as writing a book or developing a comprehensive wellness plan. Journaling aids in personal accountability and progress tracking and enables the storyteller within each individual. It allows one to trace the arc of their development, offering insights into both setbacks and advancements.

Such a practice emphasizes that progress is not always linear. By comparing earlier entries to current practices, one can identify patterns of backsliding or forward strides, gaining a clear view of their overall trajectory. This reflective practice assures that the individual will often observe some form of progress, providing motivation and evidence of the benefits of their sustained efforts.

In essence, journaling transforms individual experiences into a coherent narrative, highlighting the journey's milestones and the lessons learned along the way. This enriches the individual's understanding of their habits and needs and offers valuable insights to guide others on similar paths toward health and vitality.

DETAILED JOURNEY THROUGH RACES

As part of this ongoing documentation, it's essential to highlight the milestones achieved in various endurance sports, which have been a significant aspect of my journey. This includes participation in half marathons, triathlons, and cycling events from 2019 through April 2024, reflecting both the challenges and accomplishments.

Each table below provides detailed metrics of the various races I have participated in, including time, pace, and other pertinent details. This systematic documentation of my milestones illustrates how a transformed lifestyle has been crucial in enhancing my physical endurance and optimizing my performance across different disciplines.

Official Race Results

Run - The Chevron Marathon - 1/20/2019		
Distance	Time	Average Pace
26.2 Miles	5:49:19	14:21 / Mile

Run - The Woodlands Half Marathon - 3/2/2019		
Distance	Time	Average Pace
13.1 Miles	2:12:33	10:07 / Mile

Run - Koala Health & Wellness HalfMarathon - 10/27/2019		
Distance	Time	Average Pace
13.1 Miles	1:58:04	9:01 / Mile

Run - Chevron Houston Marathon - 01/19/ 2020		
Distance	Time	Average Pace
26.2 Miles	05:05:49	11:40 / Mile

Run - The Woodlands Half Marathon - 3/7/2020		
Distance	Time	Average Pace
13.1 Miles	1:48:11	8:16 / Mile

Cycling - Fort Bend County Cycling - 12/20/20		
Distance	Time	Average Pace
53.31 Miles	3:04:09	17.4 mph

Cycling - Fort Bend County Road Cycling - 12/22/20		
Distance	Time	Average Speed
23.72 Miles	1:09:06	20.6 mph

Cycling - Fort Bend County Road Cycling - 12/26/20		
Distance	Time	Average Speed
53.04 Miles	2:43:39	19.4 mph

Cycling - Houston Road Cycling - 1/02/21		
Distance	Time	Average Speed
51.67 Miles	3:01:14	17.1 mph

Cycling - MCC Sugarland Ride - 1/16/21		
Distance	Time	Average Speed
42.32 Miles	2:23:40	17.7 mph

Cycling - Fort Bend County Road Cycling - 1/23/21

Distance	Time	Average Speed
63.01 Miles	3:36:39	17.5 mph

Cycling - Sugarland Road Cycling - 1/30/21

Distance	Time	Average Speed
51.48 Miles	2:46:19	18.6 mph

Cycling - Missouri City Road Cycling - 2/6/21

Distance	Time	Average Speed
67.97 Miles	3:47:46	17.9 mph

Run - The Woodlands Half Marathon - 3/6/2021

Distance	Time	Average Pace
13.1 Miles	1:48:28	8:17 / Mile

Cycling - Fort Bend County Road Cycling - 3/13/21

Distance	Time	Average Speed
57.55 Miles	3:13:36	17.8 mph

Cycling - Simonton Road Cycling - 3/20/21

Distance	Time	Average Speed
61.09 Miles	3:11:34	19.1 mph

Cycling - Fort Bend County Road Cycling - 3/27/21

Distance	Time	Average Speed
29.06 Miles	1:24:11	20.7 mph

Cycling - Fort Bend County Road Cycling - 4/03/21

Distance	Time	Average Speed
48.14 Miles	2:30:40	19.2 mph

Cycling -Montgomery County Cycling - 4/18/21		
Distance	Time	Average Speed
88.28 Miles	5:30:15	16 mph

Cycling - Sugar Land Road Cycling - 4/24/21		
Distance	Time	Average Speed
47.36 Miles	2:23:30	19.8 mph

Cycling - Fort Bend County Road Cycling - 5/2/21		
Distance	Time	Average Speed
72.34 Miles	3:59:05	18.2 mph

Cycling - Fort Bend County Road Cycling - 05/8/21		
Distance	Time	Average Speed
57.83 Miles	3:06:39	18.6 mph

Cycling - Fort Bend County Road Cycling - 5/13/21		
Distance	Time	Average Speed
22.83 Miles	1:08:30	20.9 mph

Cycling - South Houston Cycling - 5/22/21		
Distance	Time	Average Speed
67.84 Miles	3:43:41	18.2 mph

Cycling - Sugar Land Road Cycling - 05/29/21		
Distance	Time	Average Speed
49.16 Miles	2:25:23	20.3 mph

Cycling - Fort Bend County Road Cycling - 05/31/21		
Distance	Time	Average Speed
46.56 Miles	2:10:59	21.3 mph

Cycling - Fort Bend County Road Cycling - 06/12/21

Distance	Time	Average Speed
44.43 Miles	2:11:24	20.3 mph

Triathlon Event - Cypress Sprint Triathlon - 07/25/21

Distance	Time	Swim	Transition 1
16.44 Miles	1:45:59	37:07:00	5:12 / 100 yards	2:32

Bike		Transition 2	Run	
36:54:00	20.7 mph	2:00	27:25:00	8:43 / Mile

Cycling - Harris County Road Cycling - 7/31/21

Distance	Time	Average Speed
51.77 Miles	2:25:58	21.3 mph

Cycling - Harris County Road Cycling - 08/21/21

Distance	Time	Average Speed
52.04 Miles	2:46:41	18.7 mph

Cycling - Harris County Road Cycling - 09/11/21		
Distance	Time	Average Speed
52.73 Miles	2:50:16	18.6 mph

Cycling - Fort Bend County Road Cycling - 09/23/21		
Distance	Time	Average Speed
24.34 Miles	1:05:37	22.3 mph

Cycling - Sugar Land Road Cycling - 10/02/21		
Distance	Time	Average Speed
55.18 Miles	2:40:17	20.7 mph

Cycling – Fort Bend County Road Cycling - 10/21/21		
Distance	Time	Average Speed
24.22 Miles	1:05:31	22.2 mph

Run - Houston Half Marathon - 10/31/2021

Distance	Time	Average Pace
13.3 Miles	1:38:09	7:22 / Mile

Cycling - Fort Bend County Road Cycling - 12/14/21

Distance	Time	Average Speed
24.68 Miles	1:13:36	20.1 mph

Run - Aramco Houston Half Marathon - 01/16/2022

Distance	Time	Average Pace
13.1 Miles	1:43:19	7:51 / Mile

Run - Katy Half Marathon - 02/12/2022

Distance	Time	Average Pace
13.4 Miles	1:48:00	8:02 / Mile

Run - The Woodlands Half Marathon - 03/05/2022

Distance	Time	Average Pace
13.1 Miles	1:48:45	8:17 / Mile

Triathlon Event - No Label Triathlon - 05/21/22

Distance	Time	Swim		Transition 1
15.40 Miles	1:10	7:56.2	3:11 / 100 yards	1:53
Bike		Transition 2	Run	
36:34.7	22.8 mph	1:14	23:34	7:52 / Mile

Run - Houston Half Marathon - 10/30/2022

Distance	Time	Average Pace
13.4 Miles	1:46:25	7:54 / Mile

Run - Aramco Houston Half Marathon - 01/15/2023

Distance	Time	Average Pace
13.1 Miles	1:41:38	7:44 / Mile

Run - Katy Half Marathon - 02/11/2023

Distance	Time	Average Pace
13.13 Miles	1:40:48	7:41 / Mile

Run - Woodlands Half Marathon - 03/04/2023

Distance	Time	Average Pace
13.13 Miles	1:39:48	7:36 / Mile

Triathlon Event - No Label Triathlon - 05/20/23

Distance	Time	Swim		Transition 1
15.40 Miles	1:10:10	8:51.5	3:59 / 100 yards	1:48.1
Bike		Transition 2	Run	
33:15:00	22.0 mph	0:58.4	25:17:00	8.29 / Mile

Run - Cypress Half Marathon - 11/12/2023

Distance	Time	Average Pace
13.11 Miles	1:43:46	7:55 / Mile

Run - The Aramco Houston Half Marathon - 01/14/2024

Distance	Time	Average Pace
13.25 Miles	1:42:27	7:44 / Mile

Run - Katy Half Marathon - 02/10/2024

Distance	Time	Average Pace
13.1 Miles	1:47:30	8.09 / Mile

Run - The Woodlands Half Marathon - 03/02/2024

Distance	Time	Average Pace
13.1 Miles	1:42:13	7.45 / Mile

Sprint Triathlon Event - MKT Sprint Triathlon - 03/16/24

Distance	Time	Swim	Transition 1
15.22 Miles	1:13:11	9:59:09	1:37.5

Bike		Transition 2	Run	
38:51:00	18.9 mph	1:05.9	21:37:00	7.26 / Mile

Run - Vintage Park Half Marathon - 04/21/2024		
Distance	**Time**	**Average Pace**
13.12 Miles	1:44:21	7.57 / Mile

These entries encapsulate the essence of each event I participated in, focusing on the raw data that reflects my growth and is physical evidence of the OMAD lifestyle's benefits. Each event is the culmination of daily practices recorded in my journals—meticulous meal planning to ensure balanced nutrition, timely hydration, and careful monitoring of physical responses. These practices have been critical in boosting my stamina and enhancing my ability to endure long distances and challenging races.

Reflecting on the Journey

Reflecting on this detailed journey through races, it becomes evident that journaling has served as a tool for self-discovery and accountability and a platform to measure the tangible impacts of the OMAD lifestyle on my athletic performance. The discipline of consistent documentation has enabled a clearer perspective on the interplay between nutrition, exercise, and overall well-being.

The routine aspect of journaling and the exhilarating challenges of races I undertook underscore the multifaceted benefits of the OMAD approach. It illustrates how an individual can harness the power of meticulous self-monitoring to enhance physical capabilities, manage dietary needs effectively, and ultimately lead a healthier, more fulfilled life.

Through these insights and records, I want to inspire others to consider how documenting their own journeys, in whatever form that may take, can profoundly impact their personal and athletic achievements.

While this section concludes, it certainly does not signify the end of my athletic journey. I am eagerly committed to continuing this adventure, constantly striving to enhance my performance and embrace new challenges.

INDIVIDUALS STARTING THEIR HEALTH AND WELLNESS JOURNEY WITH JOURNALING

For individuals embarking on a journey focused on wellness and health, journaling will serve as a key tool in cultivating your physical, mental, and emotional resilience. The simple act of documenting dietary choices, meal timing, and exercise routines and identifying their direct impacts on your overall well-being can significantly bolster your health journey.

Just as the tables in the previous section meticulously document the specifics of each milestone—time, pace, and other critical details—your nutritional journal should detail everything consumed, from main meals like breakfast, lunch, and dinner to snacks and beverages. Examples might include entries like "bagels for breakfast, rice and chicken for lunch, pizza for dinner," along with beverages such as "ginger tea" or "four 16-ounce bottles of water." Recording these details provides a comprehensive view of your dietary habits, allowing you to recognize patterns and make informed adjustments.

The documentation of races exemplifies how precise tracking of physical activities, similar to dietary logging, enhances understanding and facilitates performance improvements. Through the lens of journaling, the nuances of how small adjustments in diet and exercise contribute to overall vitality become apparent. This can inspire continued efforts and adjustments, enhancing the effectiveness of health strategies. By maintaining a record of these efforts, individuals can visualize progress and understand the interplay between various elements of their health regimen.

Ultimately, the discipline of journaling about these health-related aspects reinforces the connection between routine practices and their outcomes. It reflects the journey toward achieving a balanced state of wellness, providing a clear path to follow and adjust as needed. This detailed recording mirrors the meticulous documentation of race metrics, showcasing how each logged entry—not just in dietary terms but in all areas of wellness—contributes significantly to personal development andachievement.

8

EMPOWERING WELLNESS

AMPLIFYING THE OMAD LIFESTYLE THROUGH COMMUNITY ENGAGEMENT

In my journey with the OMAD lifestyle, the concept of community includes the tangible, real-world connections made through local meetups and groups. The aspiration to grow this support into physical spaces is evident in the initiatives undertaken through Gleanit Consulting.

Gleanit Consulting is a platform for disseminating information about the OMAD lifestyle; it is an ecosystem designed to provide comprehensive wellness tools. These tools are crafted to assist individuals in becoming physically fit, mentally clear, and emotionally stable. By integrating nutritional advice, exercise routines, and strategic fasting into a holistic approach to wellness, Gleanit aims to foster a real-world community that supports each member's health journey.

Website as a Gateway to Real-World Interactions

The website serves as the foundation for this community. The pages outline a clear, inviting path for visitors to engage with the content and eventually participate in local groups and events. Visitors are introduced to the Gleanit lifestyle, emphasizing wellness, mindfulness, and self-actualization. This sets the stage for deeper engagement through services like personalized consultations.

Strategizing Community Building through Local Meetups

The strategic approach to building local communities involves organizing meetups that provide platforms for members to share experiences, challenges, and successes. These gatherings are envisioned to be spaces where the principles of the OMAD lifestyle are practiced and promoted in a supportive, communal environment.

By fostering these local groups, Gleanit Consulting aims to inspire global change through success stories that resonate from one member to another, creating a ripple effect that enhances the visibility and viability of the OMAD lifestyle. Integrating real-life community engagement will create a robust framework for individuals to adopt and thrive within this wellness-focused lifestyle.

INSPIRING GLOBAL CHANGE THROUGH SUCCESS STORIES

The universal applicability and significant impact of the OMAD lifestyle are vividly illustrated through inspiring success stories from individuals worldwide. These narratives showcase the health benefits and the mental and emotional transformations accompanying this dietary practice.

Among the notable advocates of related practices, such as intermittent fasting, which shares core principles with OMAD, is

Dr. Andrew Huberman, a neuroscientist with a significant social media following. Dr. Huberman has discussed the potential benefits associated with delayed eating on various platforms, including his podcasts. These include improvements in cognitive function and overall mental well-being. Although Dr. Huberman's discussions are more broadly about fasting, the underlying principles align closely with the OMAD lifestyle, underscoring its benefits in enhancing mental clarity and health resilience.

Another influential figure in the world of longevity and wellness is Peter Attia, known for his deep dives into the science of longevity. While his book, "Outlive," extends beyond the scope of OMAD, his research and discussions often touch upon the benefits of strategic eating patterns, including time-restricted eating. This again parallels the OMAD philosophy, which states that the timing of meals plays a crucial role in optimizing health outcomes.

Furthermore, inspirational figures like David Goggins, known for his extreme physical endurance and mental resilience, although not directly linked to OMAD, exemplify the deep impact of disciplined lifestyle choices on personal development and physical performance. His journey offers motivational insights into how structured challenges, akin to dietary disciplines like OMAD, can forge mental toughness and physical strength.

These stories collectively highlight the versatility of OMAD and related dietary strategies, appealing to a broad audience that may include those interested in cognitive enhancement and longevity as well as individuals seeking to overcome physical and mental barriers. They demonstrate that the principles underlying OMAD are not just about nutrition but are part of a larger narrative of holistic well-being and intentional living.

As I delved deeper into these success stories, I recognized the transformative power of OMAD across different cultures and lifestyles, emphasizing its potential to foster individual and global health improvements. This exploration can inspire everyone to consider how integrating such a disciplined eating pattern into their lives could be a key step toward achieving their health and wellness goals.

THE RIPPLE EFFECT OF HEALTH TRANSFORMATION

Personal health transformations often extend their impact beyond individuals, creating ripple effects that inspire broader community changes and global health trends. Within my family, I've seen firsthand how the implementation of nutritious meal choices and regular exercise has fostered a healthier way of living. We've found ourselves largely free from frequent illnesses, headaches, and fatigue and have experienced enhanced energy levels and physical strength throughout the day.

This approach has shown us that the right foods can function as preventive medicine, helping us live healthier and more vibrant lives.

This ripple effect has also been observed in broader communities as individuals implementing such lifestyles inspire others around them. For example, when multiple people adopt OMAD or other disciplined eating habits and share their positive experiences, the impact is noticeable in the encouragement and interest it generates among friends and family. The ripple effect of health transformation leads to the creation of supportive networks where participants exchange knowledge and share practical tips, thereby enhancing the community's collective well-being.

In a global context, health movements often arise from these grassroots transformations. When people experience significant improvements in their health through lifestyle changes and share these success stories, they help popularize practices that align with emerging trends in nutrition, exercise, and holistic wellness. Whether it's by leveraging social media platforms or forming real-world groups, the ripple effect of health transformation can shape public health trends and foster a global shift toward healthier, more sustainable living.

To join this growing community and take the first step towards transforming your health and wellness, visit Gleanit Consulting today, where you can explore the resources, connect with like-minded individuals, and start your journey to a healthier, more balanced life.

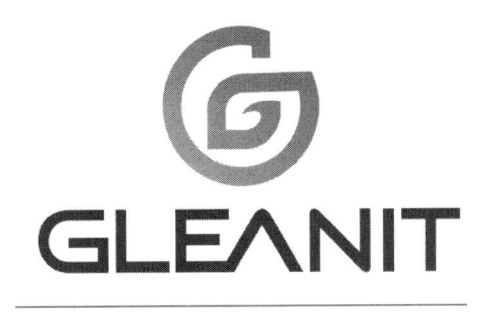

www.gleanits.com

9

GETTING STARTED

Transitioning to a one-meal-a-day (OMAD) lifestyle is a journey that demands strategic planning, sustained motivation, and perseverance. Throughout this book, we have delved into my personal journey, shared extensive advice, and celebrated various milestones. But as we move forward, it's crucial to highlight that all the knowledge and inspiration we've discussed is not intended to prescribe a one-size-fits-all method but rather to reflect on the steps I would take if I were to start this journey or advise my past self at the start of this transformative lifestyle. It's crafted as a reflective guide, directing the advice to myself and offering insights and considerations that helped me adopt and maintain the OMAD lifestyle successfully. For readers, consider this a source of inspiration from which you can select elements that resonate with your health goals and lifestyle choices.

FIRST STEPS

Beginning Your Journey

Starting your OMAD journey is about gradually transforming your lifestyle in a sustainable way.

Here's how to begin:

Gradual Lifestyle Changes

Before jumping directly into OMAD, start by focusing on your overall lifestyle. Prioritize nutritious meals, establish a regular eating schedule, and maintain discipline, even on weekends or when dining out. Make mindful choices about what you eat, ensuring each meal is balanced and nourishing.

Focus on Nutrition

Ensure that your single meal is both satisfying and nutritious. Incorporate a variety of foods that provide all essential nutrients. Aim for a balance of proteins, healthy fats, carbohydrates, and plenty of vegetables. This approach keeps you full and ensures your body receives the necessary vitamins and minerals.

Maintain Discipline

Discipline is key to successfully transitioning to OMAD. Whether you're at home, work, or out with friends and family, make consistent, healthy choices. Stick to your eating schedule and avoid the temptation to snack outside your designated meal time.

Gradual Reduction of Meals

Gradually reduce your meal frequency. If you're used to eating three meals a day, cut down to two meals, then to one and a half, and finally, to one satisfying meal. This gradual approach helps your body adjust to the new eating pattern, making the transition smoother and more sustainable. It's important to monitor your calorie intake and ensure that each meal provides sufficient nutrients to sustain energy levels and overall health, especially if you lead an active lifestyle.

This careful management of your diet will support bodily functions and physical activities effectively without compromising your well-being.

Key to Reaping OMAD Benefits: Nutritional Balance and Flexibility

Overcoming Initial Challenges with Nutritional Balance

Transitioning to the OMAD lifestyle introduces a significant shift in your dietary habits. It's not just about reducing the frequency of meals but ensuring that the single meal you consume is profoundly nourishing and satisfying. Nutritional balance is paramount in this meal to ensure it fuels your body effectively for 24 hours. This balance involves a well-rounded intake of proteins, healthy fats, carbohydrates, and vitamins and minerals sourced from vegetables and fruits.

Ensuring your meal is nutritionally complete helps mitigate common initial challenges such as fatigue, hunger pangs, and mental fog.

A well-planned meal combats these issues by stabilizing blood sugar levels and releasing sustained energy. This approach is particularly crucial during the adaptation phase when your body is still adjusting to more extended fasting periods. Proper meal composition supports this adjustment phase, making the transition smoother and more manageable.

Flexibility Within Structure: Key to Long-Term Success

While discipline is crucial, flexibility within your eating schedule can significantly enhance the OMAD lifestyle's sustainability. This flexibility allows for adjustments based on daily energy demands and social commitments, making it easier to maintain this lifestyle without feeling restricted.

For example, if a dinner with friends is planned, you might choose to make that your meal of the day. On days when you need more energy, adjusting the timing of your meal to post-exercise can help maximize nutrient absorption and recovery.

Incorporating flexibility helps address one of the major hurdles newcomers face: the rigidity of eating schedules. By allowing yourself the freedom to adjust meal times within certain limits, you can make OMAD a natural and enjoyable part of your life. This adaptability ensures that your dietary regimen complements rather than complicates your lifestyle.

The success of OMAD is not just in adhering to a fasting schedule but in the thoughtful composition of your meal and the strategic flexibility of your approach. This thoughtful planning ensures that you meet your body's nutritional needs while accommodating the realities of your everyday life. By doing so, you can turn what might seem like a daunting dietary challenge into a sustainable and beneficial lifestyle, enhancing both your physical and mental well-being.

Integrate Workouts

Incorporate daily physical activities, whether running, cycling, swimming, or hitting the gym, into your routine. Find what suits you best. Consistency is crucial. Over time, your body will start craving these workouts, and you'll find joy in staying active. Combining regular exercise and a disciplined eating schedule will enhance your overall well-being and fitness levels.

Embrace the Journey

Understand that this transformation took years. Starting with intermittent fasting and witnessing its positive impacts on physical and mental well-being, this approach can be taken further, gradually prolonging the fasting windows, experimenting with different things, witnessing significant positive changes, and finally adopting the OMAD lifestyle.

Finding the balance between diet and physical activity is a personalized journey that will significantly improve your overall well-being.

Essential Preparations: Setting the Foundation for Success

Transitioning to the OMAD lifestyle isn't just about changing how often you eat; it requires a holistic approach to both mental and physical preparation.

The first step in laying the groundwork for a successful transformation is mental preparation.

1. Mental Readiness

Understanding Your Motives

To successfully adopt and maintain the OMAD lifestyle, it is essential to clearly understand and articulate your reasons for making this significant change. Whether your motivation stems from health concerns, weight management goals, the desire for enhanced mental clarity, or a broader pursuit of overall well-being, recognizing and defining these motives will anchor your commitment and guide your journey.

Understanding and focusing on why you choose the OMAD lifestyle will help you navigate challenges and stay committed to your goals. This self-awareness fosters persistence and enhances the personal satisfaction and benefits derived from this lifestyle change.

Setting Expectations: Realistic Goals and Timelines

Setting clear and realistic expectations is crucial for transitioning to the OMAD lifestyle, both for immediate success and long-term sustainability.

Here's how you can approach this:

Define Clear, Achievable Goals

- **Start Small:** If you're new to fasting or meal reduction, gradually shorten your eating window instead of jumping straight to a single meal a day. For instance, if you typically eat over a 12-hour period, aim to reduce this to 10 hours and slowly work your way down.

- **Customize Your Approach:** Tailor the OMAD transition to your individual lifestyle and health needs. For example, if you have a physically demanding job or lifestyle, your approach to calorie intake and meal timing might differ from someone with a more sedentary lifestyle. Moreover, integrating exercise into your routine is crucial; plan your single meal to optimize energy for your workouts. For instance, you might find having your meal a few hours before your physical activity allows for peak performance.

Establish Realistic Timelines

- **Gradual Transition:** Adapting to OMAD can take several weeks to months. For example, spend the first few months focusing on reducing your eating window, adjusting the size and content of your meals to ensure nutritional adequacy, and so on.

- **Monitor and Adjust:** Regularly assess your progress. It's okay to adjust your goals as you learn more about how your body responds to the changes. For example, if you find your energy levels are depleting, you might need to adjust the nutrient composition of your meal or the timing of your eating window.

For example, a person who is used to eating every 3-4 hours might set a goal to eliminate snacks between meals first, then gradually extend the time between meals, aiming for a 6 to 8-hour eating window before transitioning to OMAD.

Likewise, an athlete might focus on timing their single meal to support their training schedule, starting with a larger post-training meal and adjusting as needed based on performance and recovery feedback.

This approach ensures that you maintain the energy and nutrients needed to support both your daily activities and any specific exercise regimen, making the transition to OMAD effective and sustainable.

Incorporating Patience into Your Plan

- **Acknowledge Adjustments:** Recognize that some days will be more challenging than others. Incorporating flexibility in your diet, such as allowing for a lighter meal or snack when really needed, can help maintain overall progress without feeling overwhelmed.

- **Celebrate Small Victories:** Each step towards narrowing your eating window is progress. Celebrating these small victories can provide motivation and a sense of accomplishment.

By setting clear, achievable goals and realistic timelines, you'll be better prepared to manage the transition smoothly and effectively, ensuring that your move to the OMAD lifestyle is sustainable and beneficial in the long term.

2. Physical and Meal Preparation

A lifestyle change requires a comprehensive approach to both physical and meal preparation. This foundational phase is about creating a supportive environment that aligns with your new dietary and fitness goals.

Organizing Your Space

Your physical environment plays a crucial role in the success of your journey. Begin by reorganizing your kitchen and pantry to remove any temptations. Clear out foods that don't align with your new eating plan, such as processed snacks and sugary treats, and make room for wholesome ingredients that support satiety and nutrition. This proactive step prevents impulsive eating and simplifies your meal preparation process.

Strategic Grocery Shopping

When shopping, focus on purchasing whole foods rich in essential nutrients. These include high-quality proteins, healthy fats, a wide range of fibers, and foods dense in vitamins and minerals. Planning your grocery list beforehand ensures that you have all the necessary ingredients for your meal, which helps maintain a balanced diet every day of the week.

Your approach should involve selecting categories like proteins, carbohydrates, fats, fruits, vegetables, and other essentials to streamline the shopping experience and ensure you're out of the store efficiently, often in under 15 minutes.

Thoughtful Meal Planning and Preparation

Investing time in meal planning is key to maintaining the OMAD lifestyle without feeling restricted or overwhelmed. Plan your meals to include a variety of nutrients, ensuring each dish is balanced and fulfilling. For instance, combining lean proteins with hearty vegetables and healthy fats makes each meal satisfying and nutritionally complete. This strategy helps manage your daily caloric intake and keeps your meals interesting.

Moreover, having the right tools at your disposal can significantly enhance your cooking experience, making it easier to stick to your meal plan. Cooking tools and appliances, such as slicers, blenders, etc., can make meal preparation both enjoyable and efficient.

3. Sustain Your Journey

To successfully integrate the OMAD lifestyle into your daily life, establish a solid routine that aligns with your meal preparation and eating schedule. Consistency is the cornerstone of making any lifestyle change a seamless part of your lifestyle. Designing a routine that complements your daily commitments will help embed these new habits more naturally into your everyday activities.

Moreover, it's equally important to stay adaptable. Life's unpredictability, including social gatherings and holiday feasts, requires a flexible approach to stay on track with your dietary goals. Strategize on ways to navigate these challenges without straying from your commitment. For instance, if attending a social event, plan how to incorporate OMAD into the occasion—perhaps by aligning your meal time or selecting foods that fit within your dietary framework, if possible.

This balanced approach of adherence and adaptability ensures that you can sustain your lifestyle change over the long term, regardless of the occasional curveball.

By following these steps, you'll be well on your way to successfully adopting the OMAD lifestyle. Remember, the journey is as much about mental preparation as it is about physical changes. Stay focused on your goals; soon, you'll experience the benefits of a healthier, more balanced life.

MOTIVATION AND PERSEVERANCE

Finding Your 'Why'

At Gleanit Consulting, we emphasize the synergy between mindful nutrition and lifestyle changes that cater to personal growth and self-actualization. Our community members often share that their 'why' is rooted in desires for longer-term health benefits and a more focused, energized living experience. What's your 'Why'?

OMAD Motivation Worksheet

Instructions: Complete the table below by reflecting on each prompt and recording your thoughts. This exercise will help you articulate your reasons and expectations, solidifying your OMAD journey.

The worksheet is found on the next page.

Note: Keep this worksheet handy and refer back to it, especially during challenging times or when you need to reaffirm your commitment. Regularly update your responses as you progress in your OMAD journey to reflect new insights and achievements.

Questions	Your Reflection
What specific health outcomes are you hoping to achieve with OMAD?	
Beyond physical health, what changes do you hope to see in your mental or emotional well-being?	
Who or what inspired you to start OMAD, and what personal aspirations do you connect with this lifestyle?	
What challenges do you anticipate facing as you transition to OMAD? What strategies do you plan to use to overcome these challenges?	
Imagine a successful day after fully adapting to OMAD. What does it look like? How do you feel about your body and mind?	
After completing this worksheet, how do you feel about your decision to pursue OMAD? Have you discovered any new insights or motivations?	

Dealing with Low Motivation

It is crucial to recognize the signs of waning motivation. You may feel a lack of enthusiasm for your usual meal prep, or the daily OMAD routine feels more like a chore than a positive lifestyle choice. Other signs include skipping planned meals out of disinterest rather than strategic fasting or finding excuses to deviate frequently from your eating schedule.

Strategies to Overcome Low Motivation

Set Small, Manageable Goals

Break your larger objectives into smaller, achievable milestones. For instance, if your overall goal is to adapt fully to OMAD within three months, start by focusing on achieving a consistent eating window each week. Alongside, manageable exercise routines should be integrated to maintain energy and health.

Change Your Environment

Sometimes, a shift in your surroundings can bring new energy to your routine. To rejuvenate your interest, arrange your kitchen, plan your meal at a different time of day, or even try eating in a new setting. Consider changing your workout location or trying new physical activities to keep your daily routine exciting.

Reward System

Establish rewards for meeting smaller goals. These don't have to contradict your diet—think about a new fitness gadget, a session with a personal trainer, or a day trip to a place where you can enjoy a long walk or hike. These rewards celebrate your progress and encourage you to continue your health and fitness journey.

Reflect on Your Progress

Regularly take time to reflect on the changes you've already achieved and how they've benefited you. Keeping a journal where you can visualize your progress and the hurdles you've overcome can be very motivating. Include notes on both your dietary and exercise achievements.

Seek Inspirational Content

Listen to podcasts, read books, or watch documentaries about others who have successfully integrated OMAD into their lives, along with a robust fitness routine. Learning about others' success can reignite your passion for your own journey.

Motivation Tracker

Create a motivation tracker in your preferred format, such as a spreadsheet or a dedicated section in your journal. This tool is designed to help you log and analyze your daily feelings about the OMAD lifestyle, understand patterns in your behavior, and proactively adjust your approach.

How to Use the Motivation Tracker:

Date: Fill out the current date.

Meal Choices Feeling: Describe your feelings about the meal choices for the day (e.g., satisfied, lacking, enjoyable).

Energy Level: Rate your energy level at the end of the day (High, Medium, Low).

Mood: Note your general mood throughout the day.

Deviations from Meal Plan (Reasons): Document any times you strayed from your meal plan and why.

Daily Exercise: Detail the type and duration of any exercise you did.

Exercise Impact on Mood/Energy: Reflect on how your exercise affected your mood and energy levels.

Date	Meal Choices Feeling	Energy Level	Mood	Deviations from Meal Plan (Reasons)	Daily Exercise & Its Impact on Mood/Energy
[Date]	[Positive/ Neutral/ Negative]	[High/ Medium/ Low]	[Mood]	[Describe any deviations and reasons]	[Type and duration of exercise and its impact on mood and energy]

Here's an example of how to integrate your daily entries into the tracker:

Date	Meal Choices Feeling	Energy Level	Mood	Deviations from Meal Plan (Reasons)	Daily Exercise & Its Impact on Mood/ Energy
05/16/24	Very satisfied with meal	High	Positive	None	30 minutes run; Increased energy, improved mood

Date	Meal Choices Feeling	Energy Level	Mood	Deviations from Meal Plan (Reasons)	Daily Exercise & Its Impact on Mood/Energy
05/16/24	Very satisfied with meal	High	Positive	None	30 minutes run; Increased energy, improved mood

This tracker will help you identify patterns or triggers that affect your motivation, allowing you to proactively adjust your approach.

Note: It's normal for motivation to ebb and flow. The key is not to get discouraged by the lows but to use them as an opportunity to reassess and rejuvenate your approach. Maintaining a balanced focus on nutrition and exercise will foster a resilient mindset that thrives on consistent, healthy habits.

Embarking on the OMAD lifestyle is about transforming your lifestyle. By understanding your motivations, preparing adequately, and developing strategies to maintain motivation, you're not just following a diet but embracing a journey toward improved health and wellness. Through this chapter, I have shared the steps and considerations that were instrumental in my journey. If you find aspects that resonate with you, consider how they might be adapted to your unique situation. As you explore any changes, it's essential to monitor your progress, make adjustments according to your needs, and, most importantly, acknowledge every achievement along your path.

CONCLUSION

Transitioning to the One-Meal-a-Day (OMAD) lifestyle is a journey that encompasses strategic planning, mental and physical preparation, and consistent dedication. Throughout this book, I've explored the various facets of adopting OMAD, including its integration with exercise, the importance of nutrition, and the personal growth accompanying this significant lifestyle change.

Starting with understanding the basic principles of OMAD, I discussed how gradual adjustments to meal frequency and composition can lead to significant health benefits. Emphasizing the synergy between diet and physical activity, we delved into how balanced nutrition supports both daily routines and intensive training schedules. Hydration, strategic fasting, and thoughtful meal planning have been my foundational elements for sustaining energy and enhancing performance throughout my journey.

Incorporating regular physical activity, such as running, cycling, and swimming into the OMAD lifestyle improved my overall fitness and mental clarity. Detailed accounts of various races and events highlighted the practical application of these principles, demonstrating how consistent training and disciplined eating habits lead to measurable improvements in my endurance and performance.

I also explored the challenges and strategies for overcoming obstacles associated with the OMAD lifestyle, addressing practical solutions like managing hunger, maintaining motivation, and navigating social dining situations. Journaling and tracking progress were emphasized as tools for self-reflection and continuous improvement, providing insights into how dietary and exercise habits influence overall well-being.

Setting realistic goals, preparing mentally and physically, and maintaining a flexible yet disciplined approach were identified as key factors for long-term success. By focusing on gradual lifestyle changes, understanding personal motivations, and celebrating small victories, the OMAD journey becomes a sustainable and rewarding path to better health.

As I close this book, consider how the principles discussed could be applied in your own life. Whether you choose to embrace OMAD or simply incorporate more mindfulness into your daily routines, the goal is the same: to live better, healthier, and with greater awareness. The journey towards health is not a one-size-fits-all but a personal path we can tailor to fit our unique needs and goals.

APPENDIX

NOTES

1: THE CONCEPT OF ONE MEAL A DAY

12   Sanvictores, T., Casale, J., & Huecker, M. R. (2023c, July 24). Physiology, fasting. StatPearls - NCBI Bookshelf.https://www.ncbi.nlm.nih.gov/books/NBK534877/.

13   Patterson, Ruth E., Gail A. Laughlin, Andrea Z. LaCroix, Sheri J. Hartman, Loki Natarajan, Carolyn M. Senger, María Elena Martínez, et al. 2015. "Intermittent Fasting and Human Metabolic Health." *Journal of the Academy of Nutrition and Dietetics* 115 (8): 1203–12. https://doi.org/10.1016/j.jand.2015.02.018.

13   Arnason, Terra G, Matthew W Bowen, and Kerry D Mansell. 2017. "Effects of Intermittent Fasting on Health Markers in Those with Type 2 Diabetes: A Pilot Study." *World Journal of Diabetes* 8 (4): 154. https://doi.org/10.4239/wjd.v8.i4.154.

13   Cienfuegos, Sofia, KelseyGabel, FaizaKalam, ShuhaoLin, Manoela Lima Oliveira, and Krista A. Varady. 2020. "Effects of 4- and 6-h Time-Restricted Feeding on Weight and Cardiometabolic Health: A Randomized Controlled Trial in Adults with Obesity." *Cell Metabolism* 32 (3): 366-378.e3. https://doi.org/10.1016/j.cmet.2020.06.018.

13   Chawla, Shreya, SpyridonBeretoulis, Aaron Deere, and Dina Radenkovic. 2021. "The Window Matters: A Systematic Review of Time Restricted Eating Strategies in Relation to Cortisol and Melatonin Secretion." *Nutrients* 13 (8): 2525. https://doi.org/10.3390/nu13082525.

13   Jordan, Stefan, Navpreet Tung, Maria Casanova-Acebes, Christie Chang, Claudia Cantoni, Dachuan Zhang, Theresa H. Wirtz, et al. 2019. "Dietary Intake Regulates the Circulating Inflammatory Monocyte Pool." *Cell* 178 (5):1102-1114.e17.
https://doi.org/10.1016/j.cell.2019.07.050.

13-16   Casale, Jarett, and Martin R. Huecker. 2020. "Fasting." PubMed. Treasure Island (FL): StatPearls Publishing. 2020.
https://www.ncbi.nlm.nih.gov/books/NBK534877/.

14-15   Meessen, Emma C. E., Håvard Andresen, Thomas van Barneveld, Anne van Riel, Egil I. Johansen, Anders J. Kolnes, E. Marleen Kemper, et al. 2021."Differential Effects of One Meal per Day in the Evening on Metabolic Health and Physical Performance in Lean Individuals." *Frontiers in Physiology* 12: 771944. https://doi.org/10.3389/fphys.2021.771944.

15	"REGULATION of FAT METABOLISM during EXERCISE." n.d. Gatorade Sports Science Institute. https://www.gssiweb.org/sports-science-exchange/article/regulation-of-fat-metabolism-during-exercise.
15	BaHammam, Ahmed S, and RoufPirzada. 2023. "Timing Matters: The Interplay between Early Mealtime, Circadian Rhythms, Gene Expression, Circadian Hormones, and Metabolism—a Narrative Review." *Clocks & Sleep* 5 (3): 507–35. https://doi.org/10.3390/clockssleep5030034.
15	Ho, K Y, J D Veldhuis, M L Johnson, R Furlanetto, W S Evans, K G Alberti, and M O Thorner. 1988. "Fasting Enhances Growth Hormone Secretion and Amplifies the Complex Rhythms of Growth Hormone Secretion in Man." *Journal of Clinical Investigation* 81 (4): 968–75. https://www.ncbi.nlm.nih.gov/pmc/articles/PMC329619/
15	Norrelund, H., K. S. Nair, J. O. L. Jorgensen, J. S. Christiansen, and N. Moller. 2001. "The Protein-Retaining Effects of Growth Hormone during Fasting Involve Inhibition of Muscle-Protein Breakdown." *Diabetes* 50 (1): 96–104. https://doi.org/10.2337/diabetes.50.1.96.
15	Elesawy, Basem H., Bassem M. Raafat, Aya Al Muqbali, Amr M. Abbas, and Hussein F. Sakr. 2021. "The Impact of Intermittent Fasting on Brain-Derived Neurotrophic Factor, Neurotrophin 3, and Rat Behavior in a Rat Model of Type 2 Diabetes Mellitus." *Brain Sciences* 11 (2). https://doi.org/10.3390/brainsci11020242.

16	Sedwick, Caitlin. 2012. "Yoshinori Ohsumi: Autophagy from Beginning to End." *The Journal of Cell Biology* 197 (2): 164–65. https://doi.org/10.1083/jcb.1972pi.
16	Shabkhizan, Roya, SanyaHaiaty, Marziyeh Sadat Moslehian, AhadBazmani, FatemehSadeghsoltani, HesamSaghaeiBagheri, Reza Rahbarghazi, and EbrahimSakhinia. 2023. "The Beneficial and Adverse Effects of Autophagic Response to Caloric Restriction and Fasting." *Advances in Nutrition* 14 (5): 1211–25. https://doi.org/10.1016/j.advnut.2023.07.006.
15-16	Wilhelmi de Toledo, Françoise, FranziskaGrundler, Audrey Bergouignan, Stefan Drinda, and Andreas Michalsen. 2019. "Safety, Health Improvement and Well-Being during a 4 to 21-Day Fasting Period in an Observational Study Including 1422 Subjects." Edited by MassimilianoRuscica. *PLOS ONE* 14 (1): e0209353. https://doi.org/10.1371/journal.pone.0209353.
16	Herz, Daniel, Sandra Haupt, Rebecca T Zimmer, Nadine Wachsmuth, Janis Schierbauer, Paul Zimmermann, Thomas Voït, et al. 2023. "Efficacy of Fasting in Type 1 and Type 2 Diabetes Mellitus: A Narrative Review." *Nutrients* 15 (16): 3525–25. https://doi.org/10.3390/nu15163525.
16	Teng, NurIslamiMohdFahmi, SuzanaShahar, NorFadilah Rajab, Zahara Abdul Manaf, MohamadHanapiJohari, and Wan Zurinah Wan Ngah. 2013. "Improvement of Metabolic Parameters in Healthy Older Adult Men Following a Fasting Calorie Restriction Intervention." *The Aging Male* 16 (4): 177–83. https://doi.org/10.3109/13685538.2013.832191.

17 Longo, Valter D., and Mark P. Mattson. 2014. "Fasting: Molecular Mechanisms and Clinical Applications." *Cell Metabolism* 19(2):181–92. https://doi.org/10.1016/j.cmet.2013.12.008.

2: GROWTH MINDSET: IMPLEMENTING INCREMENTAL CHANGES

18 Muscella, Antonella, Erika Stefàno, Paola Lunetti, LoredanaCapobianco, and Santo Marsigliante. 2020. "The Regulation of Fat Metabolism during Aerobic Exercise." *Biomolecules* 10 (12): 1699. https://doi.org/10.3390/biom10121699.

19 Arlinghaus, Katherine R., and Craig A. Johnston. 2018. "The Importance of Creating Habits and Routine." *American Journal of Lifestyle Medicine* 13 (2): 142–44. https://doi.org/10.1177/1559827618818044.

25 Casale, Jarett, and Martin R. Huecker. 2020. "Fasting." PubMed. Treasure Island (FL): StatPearls Publishing. 2020. https://www.ncbi.nlm.nih.gov/books/NBK534877/

25 Meessen, Emma C. E., Håvard Andresen, Thomas van Barneveld, Anne van Riel, Egil I. Johansen, Anders J. Kolnes, E. Marleen Kemper, et al. 2021. "Differential Effects of One Meal per Day in the Evening on Metabolic Health and Physical Performance in Lean Individuals." *Frontiers in Physiology* 12: 771944. https://doi.org/10.3389/fphys.2021.771944

25 Ming Yi Liu, and Shung-Quan Chen. 2022. "Effects of Low/Medium-Intensity Exercise on Fat Metabolism after

25 a 6-h Fast." *International Journal of Environmental Research and Public Health* 19 (23): 15502–2. https://doi.org/10.3390/ijerph192315502.

25 Jeukendrup, Asker. 2014. "A Step towards Personalized Sports Nutrition: Carbohydrate Intake during Exercise." *Sports Medicine* 44 (S1): 25–33. https://doi.org/10.1007/s40279-014-0148-z. pg. 24

25 Muscella, Antonella, Erika Stefàno, Paola Lunetti, LoredanaCapobianco, and Santo Marsigliante. 2020. "The Regulation of Fat Metabolism during Aerobic Exercise." *Biomolecules* 10 (12): 1699. https://doi.org/10.3390/biom10121699.

25 "REGULATION of FAT METABOLISM during EXERCISE." n.d. Gatorade Sports Science Institute.https://www.gssiweb.org/sports-science-exchange/article/regulation-of-fat-metabolism-during-exercise.

3: NUTRITION AND MEAL PLANNING

43 Jeukendrup, Asker. 2014. "A Step towards Personalized Sports Nutrition: Carbohydrate Intake during Exercise." *Sports Medicine*44 (S1): 25–33.https://doi.org/10.1007/s40279-014-0148-z.

4: THE ROLE OF EXERCISE

57   Kanaley, Jill A., Sheri R. Colberg, Matthew H. Corcoran, Steven K. Malin, Nancy R. Rodriguez, Carlos J. Crespo, John P. Kirwan, And Juleen R. Zierath. 2022. "Exercise/Physical Activity in Individuals with Type 2 Diabetes: A Consensus Statement from the American College of Sports Medicine." *Medicine & Science in Sports & Exercise* 54 (2): 353–68.https://doi.org/10.1249/mss.0000000000002800

57   Wu, Nana, Shannon S. D. Bredin, Veronica K. Jamnik, Michael S. Koehle, Yanfei Guan, Erin M. Shellington, Yongfeng Li, Jun Li, and Darren E. R. Warburton. 2021. "Association between Physical Activity Level and Cardiovascular Risk Factors in Adolescents Living with Type 1 Diabetes Mellitus: A Cross-Sectional Study." *Cardiovascular Diabetology* 20 (1).https://doi.org/10.1186/s12933-021-01255-0.

58   Thyfault, John P., and Audrey Bergouignan. 2020. "Exercise and Metabolic Health: Beyond Skeletal Muscle." *Diabetologia* 63 (8): 1464–74. https://doi.org/10.1007/s00125-020-05177-6.

58   Greer, Beau Kjerulf, Julie O'Brien, Lyndsey M Hornbuckle, and Lynn B Panton. 2021. "EPOC Comparison between Resistance Training and High-Intensity Interval Training in Aerobically Fit Women." *International Journal of Exercise Science* 14 (2): 1027–35. https://www.ncbi.nlm.nih.gov/pmc/articles/PMC8439678/.

59 Franczyk, Beata, Anna Gluba-Brzózka, Aleksandra Ciałkowska-Rysz, JanuszŁawiński, and JacekRysz. 2023. "The Impact of Aerobic Exercise on HDL Quantity and Quality: A Narrative Review." *International Journal of Molecular Sciences* 24 (5): 4653. https://doi.org/10.3390/ijms24054653.

59 Alnawwar, Majd A., Meiral I. Alraddadi, Rafaa A. Algethmi, Gufran A. Salem, Mohammed A. Salem, and Abeer A. Alharbi. 2023. "The Effect of Physical Activity on Sleep Quality and Sleep Disorder: A Systematic Review." *Cureus* 15 (8).https://doi.org/10.7759/cureus.43595.

59 Anderson, Elizabeth, and GeethaShivakumar. 2013. "Effects of Exercise and Physical Activity on Anxiety." *Frontiers in Psychiatry* 4 (27).https://doi.org/10.3389/fpsyt.2013.00027.

59 Mahindru, Aditya, PradeepPatil, and VarunAgrawal. 2023. "Role of Physical Activity on Mental Health and Well-Being: A Review." *Cureus* 15 (1).https://doi.org/10.7759/cureus.33475

60 Schuch, Felipe Barreto, and Davy Vancampfort. 2021. "Physical Activity, Exercise and Mental Disorders: It Is Time to Move On." *Trends in Psychiatry and Psychotherapy* 43 (3): 177–84. https://doi.org/10.47626/2237-6089-2021-0237

60 Pinheiro, Marina B., Juliana Oliveira, Adrian Bauman, Nicola Fairhall, Wing Kwok, and Catherine Sherrington. 2020. "Evidence on Physical Activity and Osteoporosis Prevention for People Aged 65+ Years: A Systematic

Review to Inform the WHO Guidelines on Physical Activity and Sedentary Behaviour." *International Journal of Behavioral Nutrition and Physical Activity* 17 (1).https://doi.org/10.1186/s12966-020-01040-4.

60 Benedetti, Maria Grazia, Giulia Furlini, Alessandro Zati, and Giulia Letizia Mauro. 2018. "The Effectiveness of Physical Exercise on Bone Density in Osteoporotic Patients." *BioMed Research International* 2018 (4840531): 1–10. https://doi.org/10.1155/2018/4840531

60 Mahalakshmi, B., Nancy Maurya, Shin-Da Lee, and V. Bharath Kumar. 2020. "Possible Neuroprotective Mechanisms of Physical Exercise in Neurodegeneration." *International Journal of Molecular Sciences* 21 (16): 5895. https://doi.org/10.3390/ijms21165895.

60 Sujkowski, Alyson, Luke Hong, R.J. Wessells, and Sokol V. Todi. 2022. "The Protective Role of Exercise against Age-Related Neurodegeneration." *Ageing Research Reviews* 74 (February): 101543. https://doi.org/10.1016/j.arr.2021.101543.

60 Grimanesa, Silvia, and Jose E Leon-Rojas. 2024. "The Effect of Aerobic Exercise in Neuroplasticity, Learning, and Cognition: A Systematic Review." *Curēus*, February. https://doi.org/10.7759/cureus.54021.

61 Warburton, Darren E.R., Crystal Whitney Nicol, and Shannon S.D. Bredin. 2006. "Health Benefits of Physical Activity: The Evidence." *Canadian Medical Association Journal* 174 (6): 801–9. https://doi.org/10.1503/cmaj.051351.

61	Kokkinos, Peter. 2012. "Physical Activity, Health Benefits, and Mortality Risk." *ISRN Cardiology* 2012 (718789): 1–14. https://doi.org/10.5402/2012/718789.
61	Song, S., Lee, E., & Kim, H. (2022b). Does exercise affect telomere Length? A Systematic Review and Meta-Analysis of Randomized Controlled Trials.Medicina, 58(2), 242. https://doi.org/10.3390/medicina58020242
68	Tiller, Nicholas B., Justin D. Roberts, Liam Beasley, Shaun Chapman, Jorge M. Pinto, Lee Smith, Melanie Wiffin, et al. 2019. "International Society of Sports Nutrition Position Stand: Nutritional Considerations for Single-Stage Ultra-Marathon Training and Racing." *Journal of the International Society of Sports Nutrition* 16 (1).https://doi.org/10.1186/s12970-019-0312-9

GLOSSARY

Term	Definition
OMAD	One Meal a Day is a dietary practice involving consuming only one meal per day, typically part of an intermittent fasting protocol.
Intermittent Fasting	A dietary regimen that cycles between periods of fasting and eating, aiming to time meals to allow for more extended fasting periods.
Ketosis	A metabolic state characterized by the elevation of ketones in the body, which occurs when fat provides most of the fuel for the body, typically induced by a significant reduction in carbohydrate intake or prolonged fasting.
Autophagy	A natural, regulated mechanism of the cell that removes unnecessary or dysfunctional components, allowing the orderly degradation and recycling of cellular components. It is significant during fasting and can

Term	Definition
	contribute to cell health and longevity.
Mental Clarity	Enhanced clearness of thought and cognition is often reported by individuals practicing OMAD or intermittent fasting due to reduced insulin spikes and stable blood sugar levels.
Insulin	A hormone produced in the pancreas that regulates the amount of glucose in the blood. A lack of insulin or an inability to respond to insulin can lead to diabetes. OMAD can influence insulin sensitivity and effectiveness.
Glycogen	The stored form of glucose, housed primarily in liver and muscle cells, and used as a form of energy during fasting or increased physical activity.
Ketone Bodies	Chemicals produced in the liver when there isn't enough insulin in the body to turn sugar (or glucose) into energy. They are used as an alternative energy source when glucose is not available.
Nutritional Balance	Ensuring that a diet includes an appropriate amount of all essential nutrients (proteins, fats, carbohydrates, vitamins, and minerals) to support overall health without excess or deficiency.
Fasting Window	The period during which no food is consumed. For OMAD, this typically extends for 23+ hours, with only one meal breaking the fasting period each day.
Eating Window	The designated period during which all daily food intake occurs, which is typically limited to a specific

GLOSSARY

Term	Definition
	number of hours in intermittent fasting protocols like OMAD.
Metabolic Health	Refers to the status of metabolic functions tied to the risk of cardiovascular disease and type II diabetes, among other health conditions. It typically involves factors such as blood glucose levels, cholesterol levels, blood pressure, and body composition.
Hydration	The process of providing adequate fluids to the body to ensure physiological processes operate optimally. It is crucial during fasting to prevent dehydration.
Mindfulness	A mental state achieved by focusing one's awareness on the present moment, often used as a therapeutic technique to enhance focus and reduce stress. It can be particularly helpful in managing eating habits and recognizing body signals such as hunger or fullness during OMAD.

INDEX

Adaptability, 14, 39, 40, 48, 52, 54, 64, 130, 135

Athletic Performance, 51-53, 77, 93, 101, 120

Autophagy, 16, 145

Behavioral Change, 19

Blood Sugar Levels, 12, 13, 61, 129

Calorie Intake, 7, 128, 132

Challenges; Challenges in OMAD, 2, 12, 16, 88, 89; Challenges in

Physical Activities, 4, 15, 21, 28, 67, 69, 79, 119, 124; Troubleshooting challenges, 100

Cholesterol, 57-58, 147

Cognitive Function, 17, 20, 31, 58-59, 124

Complex Carbohydrates, 21, 34-35, 89

Dietary Adjustments; Timing, 6-8, 18, 31, 33, 34, 55, 88, 90, 91

Meal Planning, 31, 34, 38-40, 41, 57, 58, 157

INDEX

Discipline; Discipline in Eating, 7, 14, 80, 81, 152

Eating Window, 8, 9, 54-55, 132-133, 138, 147

Energy Levels, 9, 14, 16, 17, 25, 29, 66, 80, 102

Exercise Routines;

Importance in OMAD, 56, 81, 83, 86, 97, 161

Documented Exercise Routines, 101-104

Fasting;

Strategic fasting, 4, 62, 63, 122, 138, 142; Types, 1, 2, 7, 9, 11, 12, 14, 16, 91, 115

Flexibility in Diet, 9, 40-46, 54, 55, 88, 99, 129, 156

Goals; Setting and Achieving, 19, 23-30, 154

Glycogen, 12, 24, 25, 146

Half marathons, 3, 4, 7, 15, ,64, 66, -79, 93, 94, 106

Health Benefits of OMAD, 8-13, 38, 41, 56, 60, 80

Historical Perspectives on Fasting, 8-12

Human Growth Hormone (HGH), 16

Incremental Progress, 28-29

Insulin, 11-17, 60, 146

Introduction, 1

Intermittent Fasting, 1, 2, 8-12, 86, 124, 130, 145

Journaling, Tracking OMAD progress: 96-105, 119-121

Ketosis, Role in fat burning during OMAD: 12, 145

Macronutrients, 30, 34, 52, 89

Mental Clarity, 1-21, 31-32, 56-61, 146

Mental Preparation, 19, 21, 131, 135

Micronutrient, 31-37, 48

Mindfulness, 60, 95, 123, 143, 147

Motivations, 18, 78, 98, 141

Nutritional Balance, 41-47, 54, 100, 129, 146

Nutritional Completeness, 13, 53

Nutritional Guidelines, 33

OMAD Principles, 48, 52, 53, 91

OMAD Benefits, 13, 16, 92

Patience and Persistence, 19, 21, 22, 99

Physical Preparation, 22, 142

Pre-Race Nutrition, 50-51

Primal Diet, 10

Quality of life, 19, 32, 57

Races; Half marathons, triathlons, cycling, 106-119

Scientific Research Support, 24

Self-Actualization, 95, 123, 136

SMART Goals, 26

Sports Disciplines, 51

Streamlining Meal Preparations, 38-39

Sustainability, 27, 78, 89, 129, 132

Time-Restricted Eating, 7, 124

Training; Physical training, 94; Marathon training, 13; Strength training, 4, 9; Sports training, 15; Training Regimen, 70-71

Transition to OMAD, 133

Type II Diabetes, 57, 61, 147

Vegetarian Diet Option, 36; Vegetarian Diet, 78, 79, 92

Wellness goals,18, 27, 52, 125

Wholesome Foods, 32, 39

Made in the USA
Columbia, SC
29 July 2024

c2e0dea5-0c32-4435-9385-d6e91a5acbceR02